COMBAT NECK PAIN

BY KARIN V. DRUMMOND, DC

COMBAT NECK PAIN

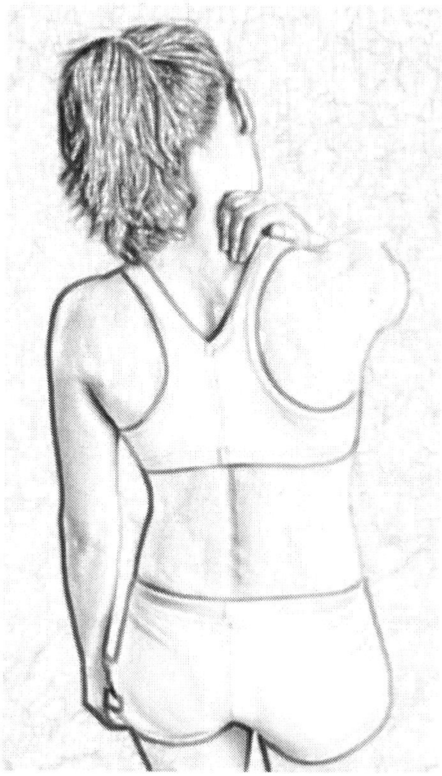

For those who suffer from neck pain, neck injury, disc degeneration, disc herniation, disc bulging, muscle tension, and more…

BY KARIN V. DRUMMOND, D.C.

Published by Blooming Ink Publishing, LLC

4712 East State Road 46
Bloomington, IN 47401

FIRST EDITION

ISBN: 978-1-943753-17-8

Library of Congress Number: 2016916841

Combat Dis-Ease Series 8

A special thank you to:

My husband, for being awesome at everything, supporting me in all my endeavors and for adjusting me as often as I need.
My prolific and published daughter, who infected me with the writings bug at the tender age of 9 years old.
My son, for trying out new things with me.
My patients, for giving as well as receiving wellness
And thank you to countless others…

Acknowledgments

Rob Schroeder, DC, president of Indy Health and Fitness and developer of the Innate Sleep Orthopedic Sleep Systems
Stanley Stanbridge, DC, inventor of the Rapid Release Technology
Jennifer Stone, BS, LAc, Editor in Chief for *Meridians: The Journal of Acupuncture and Oriental Medicine*, and owner of East West Acupuncture Inc.
Stephanie Smith, LMT, owner of Custom Massage Works
Foot Levelers, Inc, the world's leading provider of individually designed functional orthotics and therapeutic products

May this book help you navigate the waters of conflicting information on how to live pain free and well.

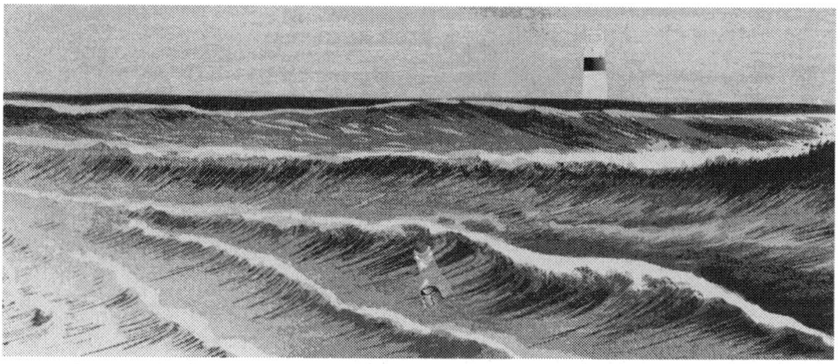

Other books by Dr. Karin Drummond:

- **Top Seven Ways to Combat the Effects of Sitting**
- **Combat Slouching**
- **Combat Headaches**
- **Combat Irritable Bowels**
- **Whiplash: More Than Just Neck Pain**
- **Whiplash to Wellness: A Chiropractor's Journey**
- **Combat Jaw Pain**

Upcoming books

- **Combat Low Back Pain**
- **Combat Foot Pain**
- **Combat Insomnia**
- and many more…

Preface

Dear Reader,

I assume that because you bought this book, you or a loved one is suffering with neck pain. Rest assured, I am writing this book for you.

I was inspired to write my books after experiencing disc herniations in my neck after a car crash. As a chiropractor, I have had plenty of experience treating neck pain. What I was not prepared for was the level of pain I experienced. I have always been sympathetic to people reporting pain, but now I am empathetic.

I've written this book to share my personal story as well as other cases of neck pain. I also offer the medical advice I give my patients. I list warning signs that your neck pain could be a sign of a serious condition, suggest treatments to consider, provide exercises and stretches to help recovery, and give advice on how to get better despite any odds.

We are all individuals with unique conditions and needs, so I advise that you seek professional care, not just from one provider, but a village of health care providers, before following any advice in this book.

I sincerely wish you and/or your loved one's wellness and a speedy recovery.

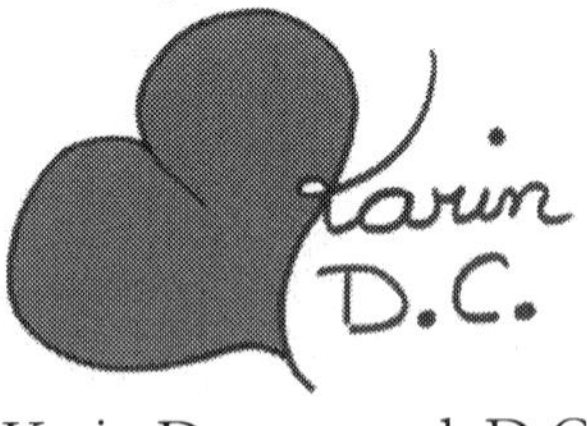

Karin Drummond, D.C.
Carin' for your health

Dr. Karin's Definition of Dis-Ease

Dis-ease is a state of being that results when a person is under prolonged stress, independent of whether it is a physical or mental stressor. Simply, it is a state of agitation and non-relaxation.

The human body evolved to handle physical stress: You either survive or you die. For example, if you get attacked by a tiger, your body automatically goes through steps to decide whether to fight or flee. Your adrenaline kicks in, activated by your fight-or-flight sympathetic nervous system.

Blood flows out of your internal organs and into your arms and legs. This rerouting of energy and blood gives you extra strength and endurance, and decreases the amount of blood loss you would experience from your organs if you were to be wounded. Your primitive brain automatically controls all of this; you don't even think about it. Your only job is to act and survive.

The primitive brain cannot tell the difference between a mental and a physical stressor. Its reaction is the same: to prepare your body for fight or flight. But if your stressor is the result of your job or an argument with a loved one, the primitive brain's fight-or-flight response is disproportional to the threat of the stressor. Your body is prepared to move, but instead you sit, tense. This is unhealthy over time because the lymphatic system (the body's sewage system) requires movement to drain the metabolic waste out of your tissues.

If the muscles stay tense, they not only prevent lymphatic drainage, but also impair blood flow to the very muscles being contracted. These constantly contracting muscles produce metabolic waste (lactic acid) and need the oxygen-filled blood to be able to contract, yet they are blocking the very flow of fluids that brings in their nutrients and drains their waste.

This sitting tense and stressed out is unhealthy over time because it leads to the buildup of toxins in the body. This is one reason why stressed people tend to be tender to touch. If your neck and upper back are stuck in chronic contraction, your muscles will become so filled with metabolic waste that they will be just plain sore, never mind sore to touch.

TENSION LEADS TO NECK PAIN!

Prolonged stress leads to adrenal fatigue; if you need a boost of energy, your body just doesn't have it to give to you. Your digestive system suffers from the diminished blood supply (because the fight-or-flight response has diverted blood away from internal organs). Then your appetite changes as you become deficient in nutrients within the intestines, leading to either weight gain or excessive weight loss.

Your blood pressure also goes up as a result of oversupplying blood to your extremities for the anticipated fight or flight. Over time, your arteries harden from being under such high pressure in a low-nutrient environment.

Eventually, your body starts deteriorating, becoming more susceptible to sickness. Every day your body fights viruses, bacteria, and fungi as well as mutations in a few of your one hundred trillion cells. It starts to lose these battles when weakened by stress, thus becoming more susceptible to colds, allergies, flu viruses, infections, cancer, and other grave diseases.

Stress is the number one cause of death; it's just given names like heart attack, cancer, stroke, suicide, etc.

This book addresses neck pain, a symptom of being in a dis-eased state. Learn how stress and lifestyle affect your neck pain.

This book and my other books contain advice on how to break this vicious cycle of stress, which leads to pain, a sign of "dis-ease," which in turn can lead to physical disease and, potentially, an early death.

BE AT EASE,
AVOID DIS-EASE.

Table of Contents

Chapter 1: MY PERSONAL STORY

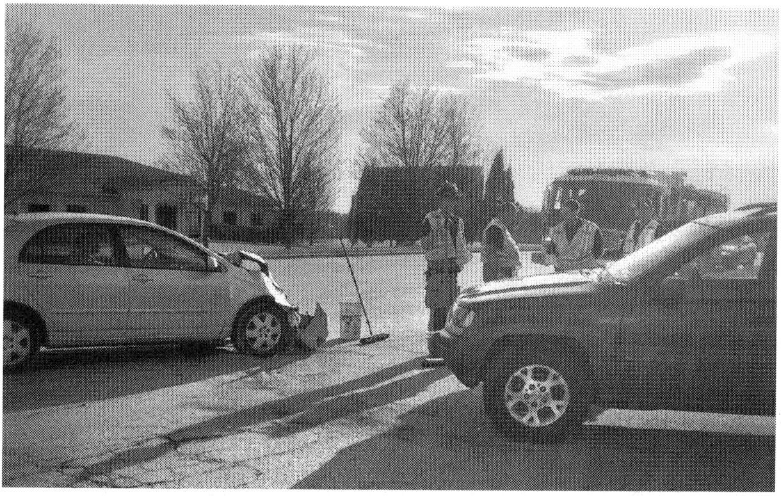

Figure 1-1: My car and the SUV
(now facing my car after spinning 180 degrees).

I WAS INVOLVED IN A CAR CRASH in 2014. As I was driving in clear weather conditions, a vehicle came out of nowhere and entered the intersection right in front of me. My instincts took over, and I slammed on the brakes, despite having no time to stop. I T-boned the other vehicle hard. You can see the aftermath of the crash in Figure 1-1.

Up until then, I was a strong, healthy chiropractor and yoga instructor who loved to do anything outdoors. The force of the impact blew four discs in my neck. I can now say I have the pleasure of knowing severe neck pain.

The Rabbit Hole of Dis-Ease

The pain I experienced after the crash was not only something I couldn't ignore, but was crippling. Just getting out of bed in the morning would cause me to yelp with pain.

The pain was so severe that I almost succumbed to falling into the "rabbit hole of dis-ease":

- If you are tired, it is hard to think well.
- If you can't think well, you may make poor choices (eat comfort foods versus nutrient-filled foods).
- If you are nutrient deprived, you will feel more tired.
- If you are tired, it is more difficult to motivate yourself to be active and exercise.
- If you don't exercise, your body will become weaker and overweight, making it vulnerable to injuries and disease (like diabetes and heart disease).
- If your body is in pain, it is difficult to rest and/or sleep, making you more vulnerable to sickness and disease.

Can you see how easy it is to fall into this vicious cycle?

After my accident:

- I was in pain.
- I was sleep deprived.
- I couldn't do all the things I love to do, and I was

getting weaker as a result!

- I was journaling my symptoms, limitations, and treatments (incase my case went through litigation). This made me focus on my pain instead of on my improvements.
- I was starting to doubt I would ever get well…

So how do you break this vicious cycle?

Start with one of the three pegs of the triad of wellness:

- Stretch or exercise more;
- Eat and drink healthier;
- Work on sleeping better and thinking positively.

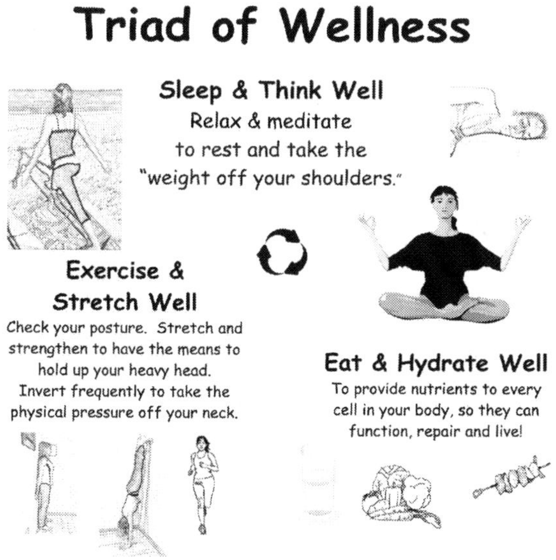

Each of these steps will bring you that much closer to wellness and less neck pain.

I started with stretching more (initially, I couldn't work on strengthening without reinjuring myself). It took hours of restorative yoga and stretching to loosen my neck up to a functional level for the day. It took months of chiropractic care and physical rehab to restore my full range of motion and reduce the pain to episodic pain versus constant severe pain.

As I healed, sleeping became easier.

When I could finally work on re-strengthening, I improved exponentially.

As a chiropractor, I was naturally sympathetic to people with neck pain; after recovering from my injuries, I also became empathetic to those with neck pain. So much so, I was inspired to write my Combat Dis-ease Series to help those beyond my local chiropractic practice.

So… What Causes Neck Pain?

You don't have to be in a crash to experience neck pain. Consider this partial list of causes:

- Poor posture while sitting, standing, or sleeping
- A worn-out mattress
- An unsupportive pillow
- Poor work ergonomics
- Repetitive stressors
- Stress (chronic, sustained muscle contraction)
- Injury
- Disease

Basically, anything that strains and compresses the neck can lead to neck pain.

Before we look at the different causes of neck pain in detail and what to do about it (specific stretches, strengthening exercises, nutritional advice, etc.), I urge you to seek the advice of a healthcare provider before trying anything I recommend in this book.

Chapter 2: WARNING SIGNS THAT YOUR NECK PAIN IS A SIGN OF A SERIOUS CONDITION

BEFORE I REVEAL how to relieve your neck pain, I must first inform you when it is imperative to seek medical attention. It would be irresponsible of me to say you could self-treat when, in fact, your neck pain could be a symptom of an underlying disease that needs medical treatment, if not immediate care.

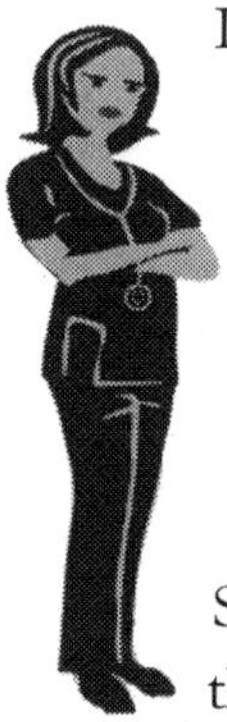

If you have a new type of neck pain; if the frequency is increasing; or if it is more intense than usual, resulting in numbness in your arm, cognitive changes, fever or any other concerning symptoms, seek immediate medical attention! It could be a sign of a more serious condition.

Seek immediate medical attention if you have any of these symptoms:

1. Neck pain with radiation down your left arm with chest pain. This can be a sign of a heart attack.
2. Neck stiffness with a fever. This could be due to infection (for example, meningitis).

I had a friend who woke up with a stiff neck on a Saturday, and it progressively worsened over a few days. He saw a medical doctor on a Thursday. The doctor prescribed muscle relaxers and pain relievers and sent him home. The next day, a friend took him to the E.R. because he appeared to be having a stroke (he was losing muscle control in his arms and legs). The E.R. doctors gave him a blood thinner. He immediately turned for the worse, and his heart stopped. Thankfully, they were able to revive him.

Soon after, the results of the blood work and scans came in. The doctors quickly realized that he had a severe infection in vertebrae in his neck. They had to remove pieces of bone from his neck to release the pressure on his spinal cord and give him mega doses of antibiotics intravenously. He was lucky to survive, let alone regain control of his arms and legs (despite the injury to his spinal cord). Any further delay of medical intervention would have resulted in death.

3. Neck pain that persists more than four to six weeks (preferably you seek a healthcare provider's advice within days if not hours, depending on the circumstances).
4. Neck pain after injury, trauma, or an accident. If this occurs, seek immediate medical attention. You may need an X-ray, CT, or MRI to rule out bone fractures or a disc herniation. It does not take a high-velocity impact to result in internal bleeding or brain injury. If you have been in a motor vehicle collision, check out my book *Whiplash to Wellness.*
5. Severe pain, numbness, tingling, or weakness down the arm. These symptoms can be a sign of a disc

herniation in your neck.

Disc herniations can be treated with chiropractic manipulation and mechanical traction, but if the herniation is grossly impinging the nerve, you may need a more immediate release of pressure on the nerve, which requires surgery.

Always get more than one opinion from at least two types of health practitioners. If you ask a surgeon how to treat a disc herniation, you are more likely to hear that you need surgery. If you ask a chiropractor, you are more likely to hear you don't need surgery. Every year, I have dozens of patients who have been told they needed surgery, and after seeing me, they were able to avoid surgery.

If you can get well without surgery, you are better off in the long run; once you have one surgery on the neck, you usually need more surgeries over time. Surgeries to the neck change the functionality of the cervical spine, leading to increased stressors to the bones above and below the surgical site. As a result, they degenerate faster, leading to another surgery. However, sometimes a condition is severe enough that the disc herniation risks the health of the nerves (which don't heal well), so surgery is imperative.

If you have any concerns about your neck pain, ask a professional's advice. You may waste a bit of time and money if no serious issues are found, but the cost of ignoring your symptoms may be far worse because it could lead to an early death.

If you suffer from neck pain and know you don't have an underlying health condition, seek the advice of a chiropractor. In my biased opinion, chiropractors are the best health practitioners to treat neck pain because they have the best tools. Plus, if they tell you need surgery, it is more likely you do need surgery because most chiropractors have the tools, training and the wherewithal to help people get well without surgery. They look at more than just your neck because your pain may be a symptom of other problems. I will discuss how other silent conditions can be the cause of your neck pain in later chapters. You can find out more about chiropractors and what they do at the end of the book.

Other practitioners who are qualified to treat musculoskeletal neck conditions are physical therapists, acupuncturists, massage therapists, and doctors of osteopathy.

To better understand what could be causing your neck pain, let's look at some basic anatomy. If you haven't seen a healthcare provider for your pain yet, the following chapters will arm you with questions you can take to your appointment.

Chapter 3: SIMPLE ANATOMY OF THE NECK

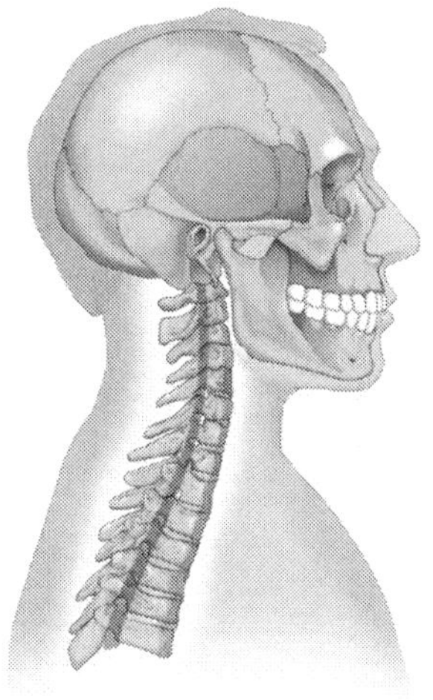

LET'S LOOK AT some basic muscle anatomy you should know if you suffer from neck pain. After you are familiar with the anatomy, you will better understand the different causes of neck pain and what you can do about it, which I cover in upcoming chapters.

The muscles I include in this chapter tend to have trigger points that can cause neck pain. (*Trigger points* are muscle spasms that put pressure on a nerve and inhibit blood flow and lymphatic drainage, which lead to pain in another area of the body.)

What follows are very basic explanations of where the muscles are and how the pain in the neck pain–inducing trigger points is caused. By knowing how these muscles are affected by your activities of daily living, you will better understand how to prevent them from tensing and be better able to massage them if they do get into a spastic state. If you want more-detailed pictures of the muscles, google the muscle names.

The Suboccipital Triangle Muscle

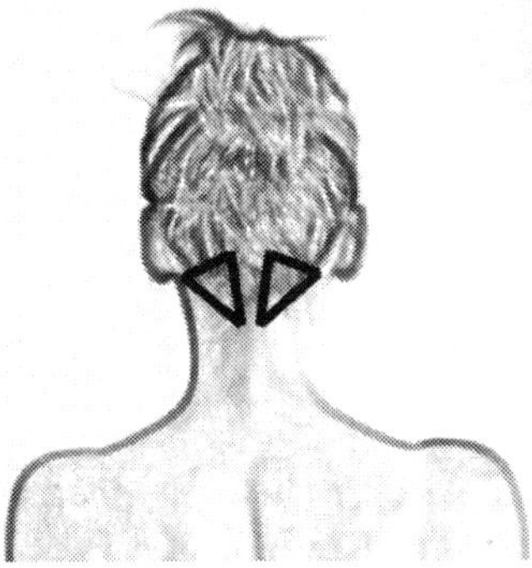

Figure 3-1

The suboccipital triangle is made up of tiny muscles that help keep the head level with the horizon as the body moves. Figure 3-1 illustrates where these muscles are located.

If you are constantly looking down with your chin out, these muscles strain to hold your head still. Chronic contraction of any muscle leads to a reduction in the flow of nutrients in and waste out, which causes metabolic waste to build up. This buildup irritates the nerves, leading to the sensation of pain, which sends aberrant signals back to the muscles to contract, resulting in trigger points. Can you see how this becomes a vicious cycle of pain that can worsen instead of improve over time?

Trigger points in these little muscles can result in neck pain and major tension headaches. If you suffer from headaches, check out my book *Combat Headaches*.

The Trapezius Muscle

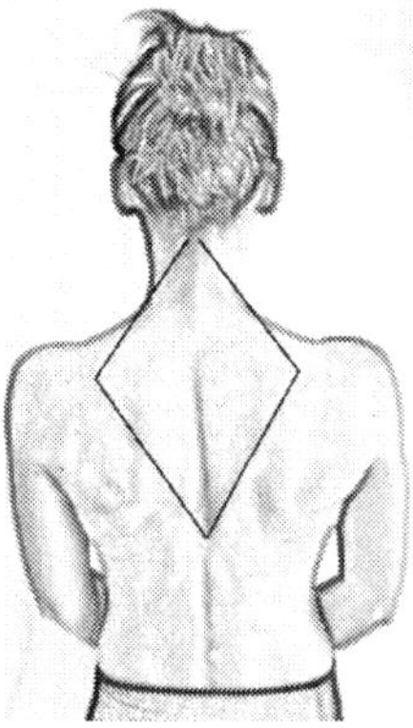

Figure 3-2

The upper half of the trapezius is the muscle that is alluded to in the phrase, "Holding the weight of the world on your shoulders."

Stress usually causes your upper trapezius to contract with tension. This results in your shoulders tightening and rising toward your ears. Figure 3-2 shows the region of the entire trapezius muscle.

Again, chronic contraction of any muscle slows the flow of blood in and the drainage of waste out. Over time, waste builds up, leading to pain in the trigger points. Trigger points in the trapezius muscle can cause neck and upper back pain.

The Levator Scapulae Muscle

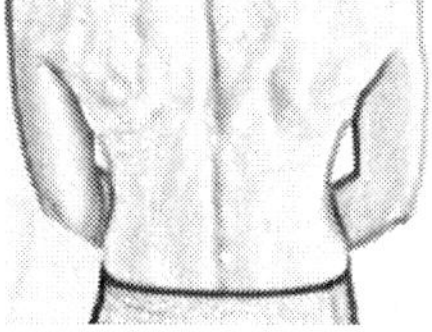

Figure 3-3

The levator scapulae are illustrated in Figure 3-3. This is another muscle that contracts when the shoulders raise up to the ears.

This muscle is under the larger trapezius muscle. It anchors onto the upper cervical spine and inserts into the upper corner of the shoulder blade. Trigger points in this muscle can cause neck pain and headaches.

The Sternocleidomastoid Muscle

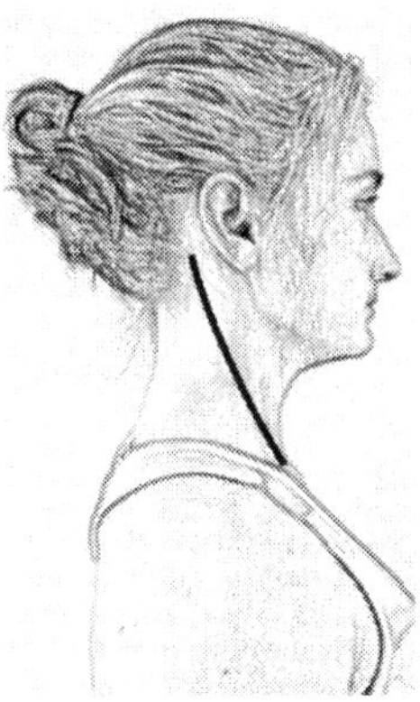

Figure 3-4

The sternocleidomastoid (SCM) is illustrated in Figure 3-4. This is the ropey muscle you should be able to see in the front of your neck.

Trigger points in this muscle can lead to pain in the jaw, head, and neck.

The Anterior Scalene Muscles

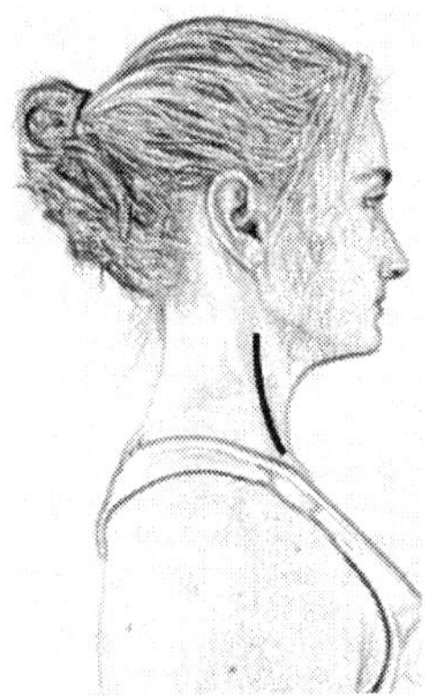

Figure 3-5

The anterior scalene muscle is illustrated in Figure 3-5. It anchors onto the neck and lifts up the upper ribs.

If you tend to breathe with your upper chest, you can strain these muscles, causing them to get overly tense and leading to pain in the trigger points that can cause neck, jaw, and head pain.

Digastric Muscles

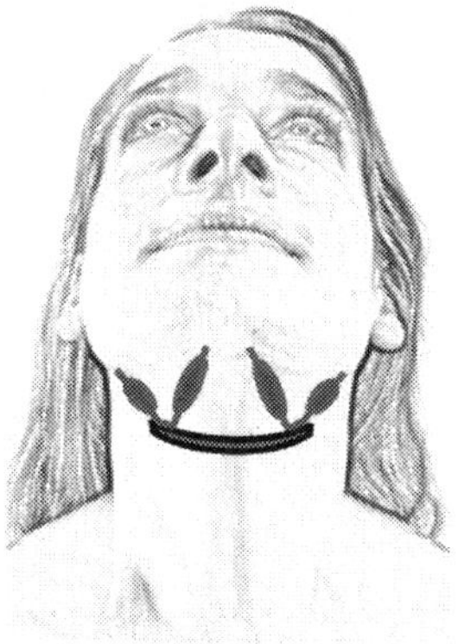

Figure 3-6

The digastric muscles are part of the submental muscles that are found under the mandible (the jawbone) as rudimentarily shown in Figure 3-6. There are more intricate muscles in this region that can be viewed under Google images. Tension here can cause neck and jaw pain.

The Omohyoid Muscle

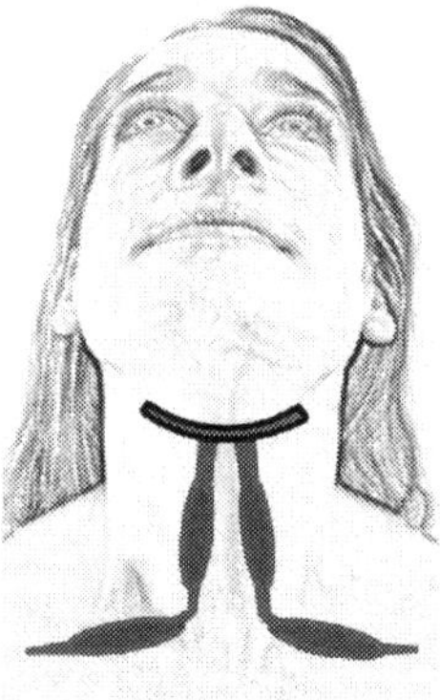

Figure 3-7

The omohyoid muscles (Figure 3-7) are just a few of the muscles in the front of the neck below the hyoid bone. They anchor to the scapula, collarbone, and neck, affecting these structures as well as the shoulders and upper back.

To complicate things further, dozens of tiny muscles orchestrate the surprisingly complicated actions of talking, chewing, and swallowing. A misfiring of any of these can result in biting your cheek, choking, or moving the jaw in such a way that it clicks or pinches its own capsule, causing it to swell and become painful.

Jaw pain can lead to neck, shoulder, and head pain. Jaw tension can mimic tooth pain, like your pain is that of a bad tooth (referred pain). If you suffer from jaw pain, check out my book *Combat Jaw Pain.*

Now let's look at the causes of neck pain.

Chapter 4: BAD POSTURE STRAINS THE NECK… ACHIEVING GOOD POSTURE AND WORK ERGONOMICS

HOLDING YOURSELF FOR ANY LENGTH of time in an abnormal unhealthy position will negatively affect the health of your spine, cause neck strain, and may also result in headaches.

Bad Posture Can Trigger Neck Pain, Headaches, Arm Pain, and Hand Numbness

Your head is like a bowling ball sitting on a golf tee. If your head weren't permanently attached, it would fall off if not balanced on top of the neck. Similarly, if your head isn't centered on your body's plumb line (i.e., the spine), your neck muscles have to strain to hold it up. This can lead to tension headaches.

What causes your head not to be centered on the spine? Bad posture. Bad posture occurs when your head isn't properly aligned over your spine and hips when you walk or sit. Slouching is a big contributor to bad posture (Figure 4-1).

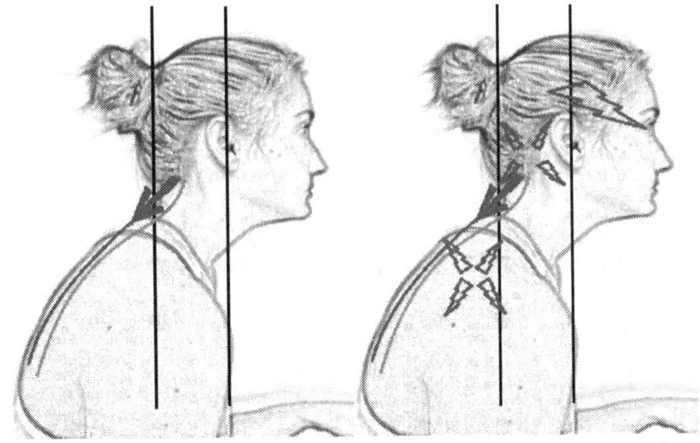

Figure 4-1: Poor posture causes neck tension, leading to headaches, pain down the arms, and/or numbness in the hands.

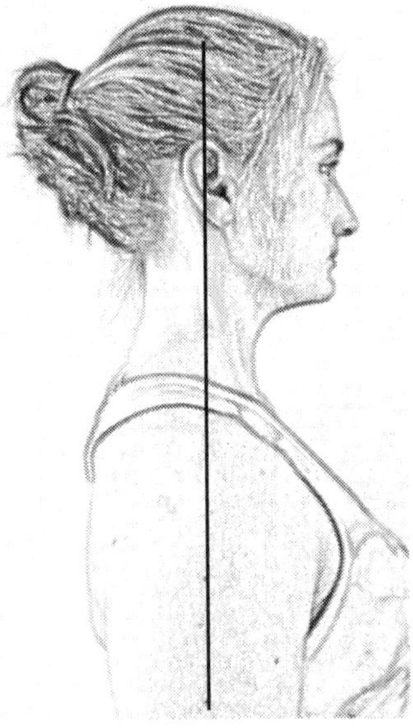

Figure 4-2: Good posture.

Maintaining good posture, as shown in Figure 4-2, is not limited to just sitting and standing. Holding items (even small ones) like smartphones, tablets, or laptops at chest level or in your lap causes you to look down for extended periods of time. Slouching strains not only your neck, but your spine, shoulders, wrists, and more.

If you find yourself standing or sitting for a prolonged period of time, keep your spine in as neutral a position as possible. When using your smartphone, hold it such that your neck remains neutral (hold it higher than your shoulder). When working on your laptop, do not put it on your lap because this encourages poor posture.

To combat chronic strain, which can lead to neck pain, move around as often as possible. It is important to move something every twenty minutes, no matter how proper your posture is. Movement gets the blood flowing, drains the lymph system, and breaks the cycle of extended muscle tension (a trigger for neck pain, back pain, headaches, and more).

To learn more about the negative effects of sitting and slouching, check out my books *Top Seven Ways to Combat the Effects of Sitting: The Silent Killer* and *Combat Slouching*.

Achieving Good Posture and Work Ergonomics

Check your posture every hour (if not more frequently). I advise patients to do this by standing with their back to the wall, with their heels, buttocks, shoulders, and back of head touching the wall (Figure 4-3). This helps verify that their ears and shoulders are aligned with the plumb line.

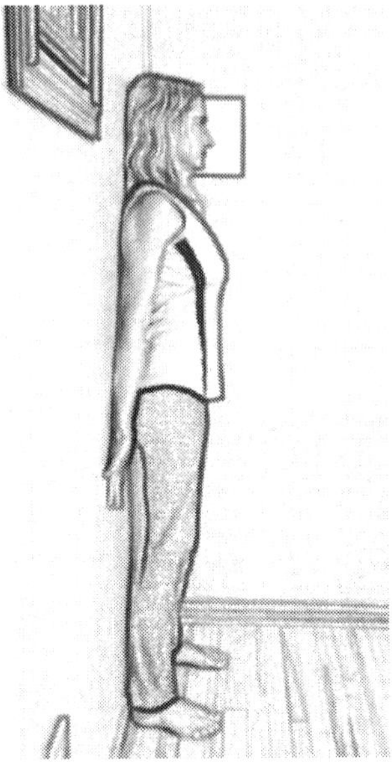

Figure 4-3: Checking your posture against a wall.

People who are chronic slouchers often find this posture check difficult to do. If you don't make good posture a habit, then you lose the ability to sit and stand up straight. As a result, your health and appearance suffer; you will develop aches and pains, and you will have a hunched back with forward rolling shoulders.

The good news is that if you practice good posture often, you will regain your ability to sit and stand up straight. (The older you are, the longer it takes, but it is still doable.) I can't tell you how many bent-over people who come to my office are able to improve over time.

To learn more about how to improve your posture, check out my book, *Combat Slouching.*

Work Ergonomics

More than half of my patients spend their days working at a desk. If it weren't for lunch and bathroom breaks, they'd never walk around. Research has proved that all of this sitting isn't good for us, but it's unavoidable for many people. If you spend hours and hours at a desk every day, it may be the cause of your neck pain.

To learn more about how sitting can cause neck pain, check out my book, *Top Seven Ways to Combat the Effects of Sitting: The Silent Killer.*

The following is what you can do to maintain good posture, reduce strain on your body, and make yourself comfortable.

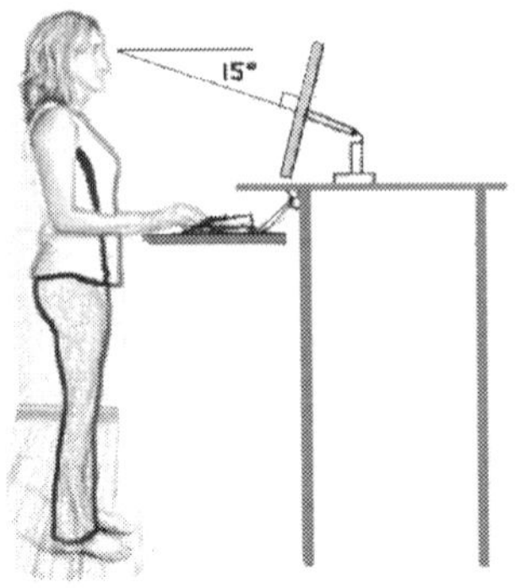

Figure 4-4: Proper ergonomics at a standing desk.

The following is advisable for both seated and standing workstations:

1. Keep your chin tucked in and head back so your ears are over your shoulders. Jutting your head forward causes your chin to tilt up so you can see what is in front of you. This posture compresses the parts in the back of your neck, including the discs between your cervical vertebrae and the nerve rootlets that run down your arms to your fingers; it also strains your posterior neck muscles. The farther your ears are in front of your plumb line (the center point of gravity), the more compression you cause. A severe slouch will compromise your whole spinal cord. Any type of pressure on your spinal cord is not good.
2. Position your monitor properly. Your eyes are "lazy" and like to tilt down about 15 degrees. If your monitor is too high, you will end up tilting your chin up so your eyes can tilt down. This too compresses the back of your neck. To combat this compression,

bring your monitor to a level such that when you tilt it back 15 degrees, your eyes naturally look at the middle of the screen at a 90-degree angle. A good computer screen should be able to tilt and swivel. The surface should be reflection free.

3. Have a window to look out of periodically to exercise your eyes. If you do not have a window in your work space, find a distant object and focus on it for a few seconds every time you leave your workstation.
4. To ensure your wrist is in a neutral position, make sure the bottom of your wrist is flat. The top of the hand will look like it is tilting up, but if you flatten the top part of your hand, you will compress the carpal tunnel, causing irritation of the median nerve, which can result in carpal tunnel syndrome (pain and numbness in the palmar aspect of the wrist, thumb, and index and middle fingers).

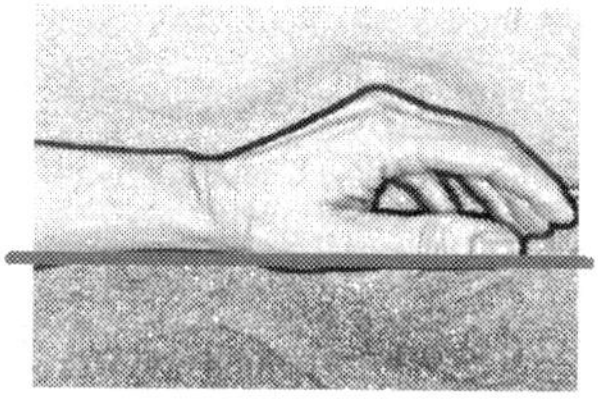

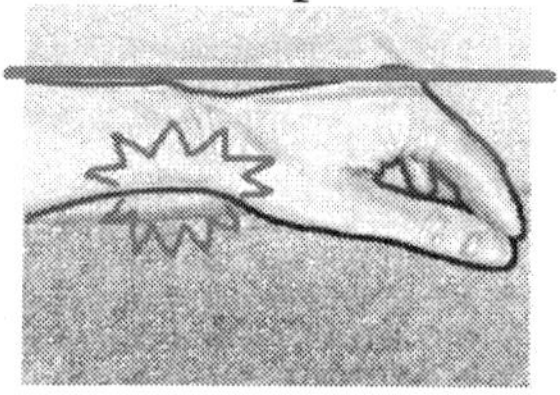

5. Place your keyboard and mouse at the proper height. Your mouse and keyboard need to be at a height that allows your lower arms to be parallel to the floor. A good chair will have an adjustable height so you can make the adjustments needed for correct arm and leg positions. A good standing desk will have an adjustable height to allow for correct arm positioning.
6. Keep your upper arm vertical with your chest open and shoulders relaxed in a back and down position.
7. If you are standing, make sure your knees are soft and

your feet are hip width apart. Wear comfortable shoes, and stand on a thick rubber mat.

The following are specific to seated workstations:

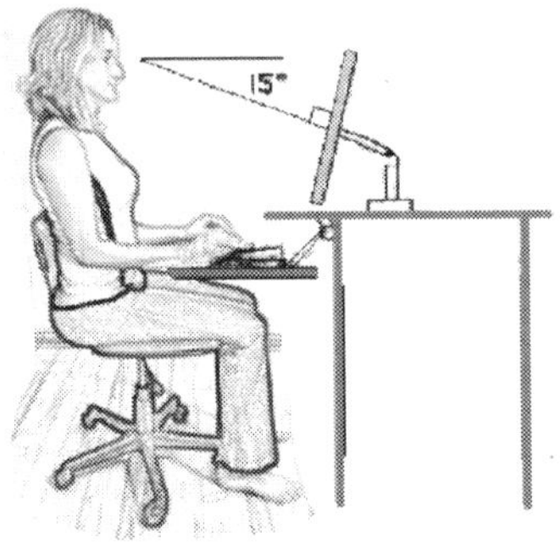

Figure 4-5: Proper ergonomics when seated at a desk.

1. Place your seat at a level that allows your knees to bend at 90 degrees and your feet to rest flat on the floor. For those who wear high heels, this is a good time to take them off. (No one will see your feet under your desk.) This is a good time to stretch your toes to help prevent bunions.
2. Make sure your lower back is supported by a lumbar support pad in the chair or a lumbar support pillow. A good chair will allow you to adjust the height and angle of the backrest to provide you with the proper support specific to your needs. If you keep a wallet or other items in your back pocket(s), make sure to take them out because they will cause a pelvic tilt that can throw your whole spine out of alignment over time.
3. Use a chair with a solid base (a five-star base if it is mobile with wheels).
4. Make sure the floor is level and flat. I have had

patients who had chronic back pain, only to find out their treatments were not lasting because the floor at their workstation was not level. They were holding their rolling chair in place all day. This strained their back muscles and constantly pulled their back out of alignment.

5. Do not sit cross-legged because it twists the pelvis, causing additional strain to the spine. It also compresses venous blood return, which potentially increases your risk of developing varicose veins.
6. Give your thighs room. Your desktop should be thin for maximum thigh space, with the keyboard in front of you.
7. Get up—preferably once an hour—and move around to get your blood flowing. Even if you just perform a mini-exercise, such as marching in place or doing some squats, any movement is good. It keeps you mentally fresher throughout the day, allowing you to work more effectively. This newfound efficiency will easily compensate for the time it takes to perform such mini-exercises.

Chapter 5: A SILENT CAUSE OF NECK PAIN… LLI AND FEET

IT'S AMAZING HOW the anatomy at one end of your body can affect the anatomy at the opposite end of your body as well as many of the body parts in between.

If you have one leg that is longer than the other, be it from growing unevenly or the result of trauma (like a fractured leg that didn't heal correctly), you may be experiencing neck pain as a result.

Leg Length Inequality (LLI)

A longer leg does not cause leg pain, but it can cause neck pain. It's like a domino effect. Standing on uneven legs causes a tilt in your pelvis (Figure 5-1). For example, if your right lower right leg is shorter than your left, your right pelvis tilts down. This causes your spine to curve to the right, and then your neck has to compensate for the spine's abnormal curvature in order to hold your head and eyes level. This creates neck pain.

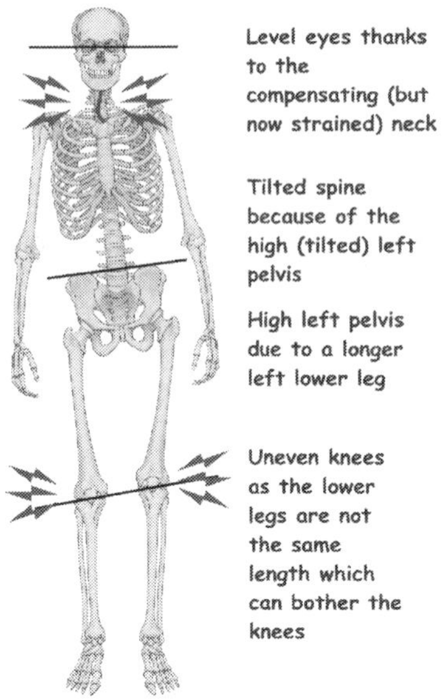

Figure 5-1: When one lower leg is longer than the other, your pelvis and back tilt to one side, and the neck curves, which can result in neck pain.

And in addition to your neck straining, your knees are irritated by walking at uneven heights.

Moving up the leg, if your left femur (thighbone) is longer than the right, this will also cause the pelvis to tilt down on the right (Figure 5-2).

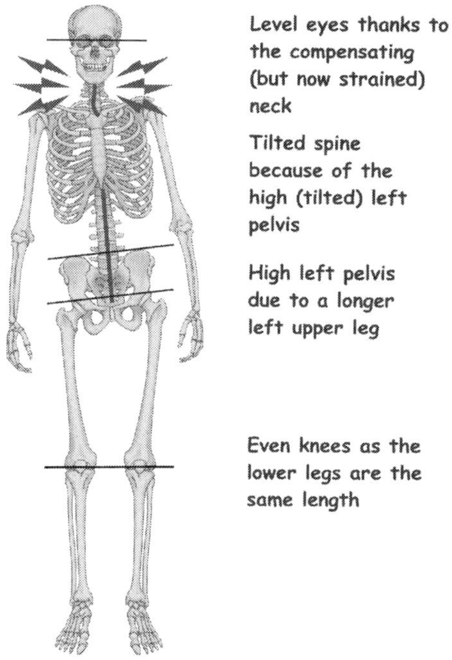

Figure 5-2: Example of a long thighbone causing a tilted pelvis, which tilts the spine, causing the neck to bend to hold the eyes level, resulting in neck pain.

But notice how the knees are even in this case. To even out your pelvis, your health care practitioner may suggest a heel lift to wear under your short leg. This helps in the first example (Figure 5-1) but would cause your knees to become uneven in the second example (Figure 5-2).

I have had many patients come in wearing a heel lift as prescribed by a health practitioner, when in fact they should not be wearing one. Let me explain further to better arm you with knowledge in case you need to explore this option with your health care provider.

Heel Lifts

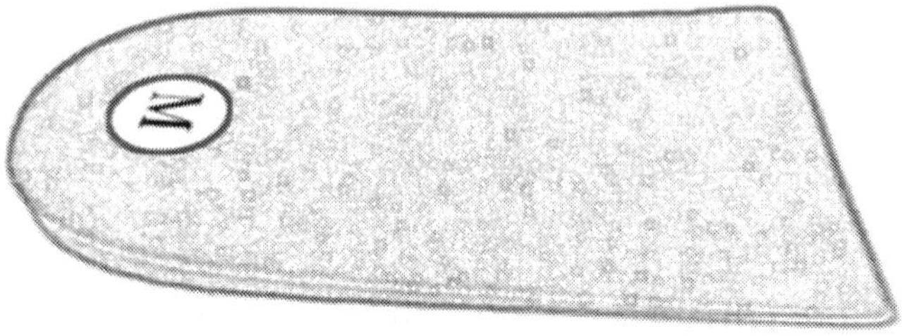

Figure 5-3: A heel lift.

Your eyes like to be level with the horizon, so to keep your head level so you can see straight, your neck has to compensate for your pelvic tilt by curving to the left (or to the right if your right leg is longer). This requires your muscles to work harder than normal to hold your head straight. This constant contraction is a strain on them. They will become tender to touch as these overworked muscles produce more metabolic waste (lactic acid) that burns.

Plus, when a muscle is held in a constantly contracted state, the lymphatic vessels are unable to drain this waste, and nutrient-filled blood is unable to flow in. This vicious cycle leads to neck pain. Over time, this strain speeds up the degeneration of the spine at these points of tension.

Checking Your Leg Length

If you have neck pain, have a chiropractor check out your leg lengths. If upon first examination it appears you have a leg length inequality, a scanogram will be ordered to verify this and to determine by how much in each bone.

If you have a true anatomical leg length inequality, only wear a heel lift if the difference is below your knees (Figure 5-4). You should feel an improvement in your neck pain (and knee pain) within a few weeks.

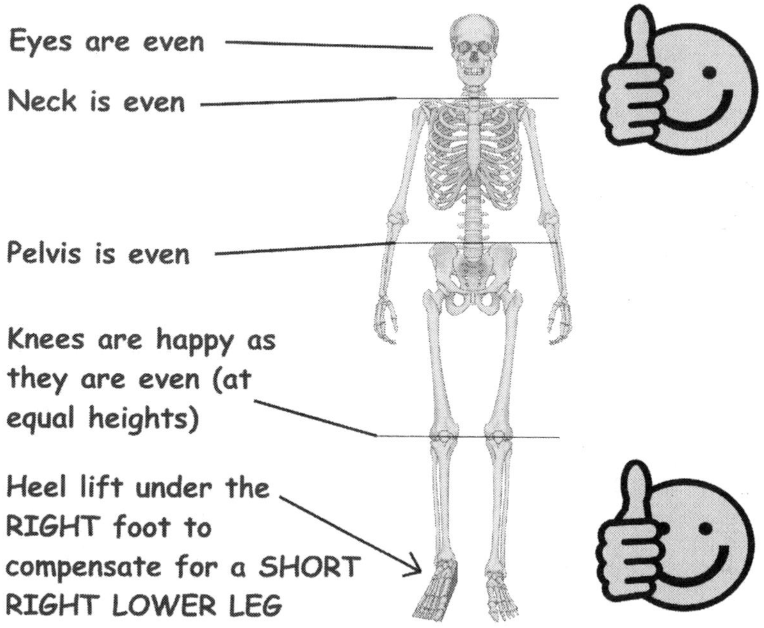

Figure 5-4: Example of a heel lift being beneficial.

If the leg length difference is in one of your thighs, wearing a heel lift can help your neck, but it will make your knees uneven, which stresses them and can speed their degeneration (Figure 5-5). You don't want to fix the original problem but create a worse one.

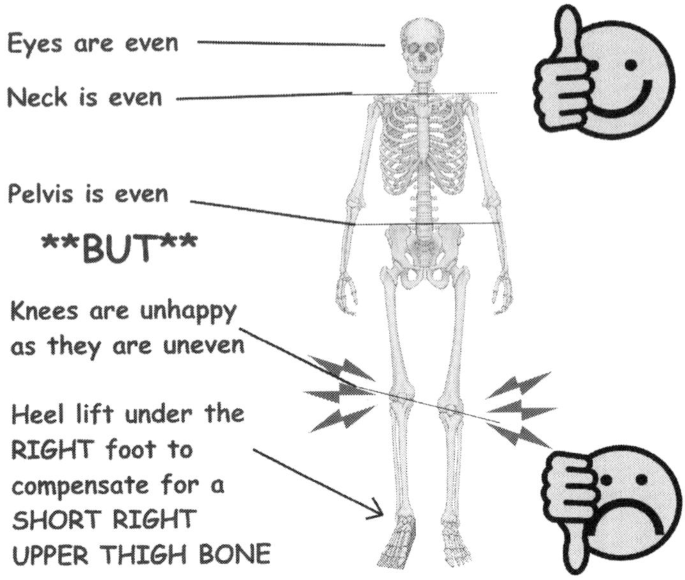

Figure 5-5: An example of a heel lift being beneficial for the neck but not for the knees.

You have the right to have both a lower and upper leg bone difference. In this case, you may need a heel lift to make your knees even, but not enough to completely level off your pelvis.

This is why it is important to talk to your health provider(s) to help determine what the best options are for you.

Collapsed Arches

If you have equal leg lengths, yet your pelvis tilts, the tilt could be caused by one foot collapsing more than the other when you walk. The foot that collapses more will cause the pelvis to tilt just like a short lower leg would.

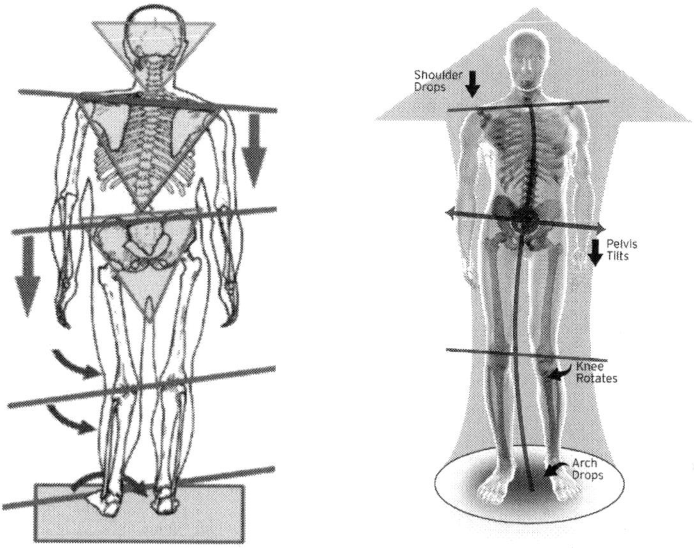

Figure 5-6: Collapsed arch causing an imbalance to the whole body. (pictures courtesy of Foot Levelers, Inc.)

Figure 5-6 shows the left arch dropping, causing the left knee to rotate, the pelvis to tilt, and the right shoulder to drop. Now the neck has to strain to keep the eyes level with the horizon by curving unnaturally.

Your pelvis can also be misaligned if your heel bone is tilted. If this is the case, you may need a wedge (Figure 5-7) to help prevent your heel from tilting.

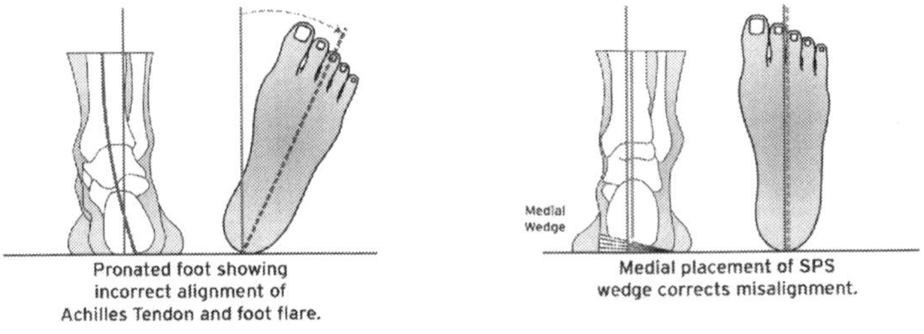

Figure 5-7: Pronated foot helping alignment of the foot.
(picture courtesy of Foot Levelers, Inc.)

The Solution

The solution for collapsed arches is orthotics. An orthotic is a supportive device you wear in your shoes to provide additional support for your feet (Figure 5-8).

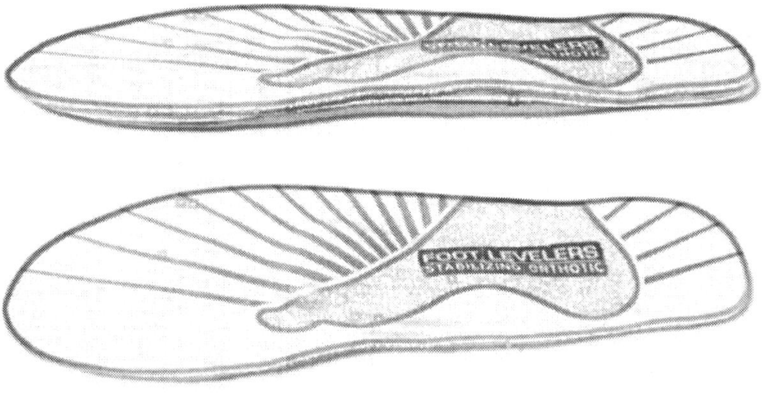

Figure 5-8: Example of orthotics from Foot Levelers, Inc.

If your treatments are not providing lasting relief for your neck pain, it may be because the foundation on which you stand is off! You may need orthotics to keep your body in alignment and to take the stress off of your neck! Otherwise, every step you take will be a strain on your neck and body.

If the arches of your feet are collapsing, this will also strain your knees. So, wearing orthotics will also help your knees! Orthotics decrease the amount of stress on knees that lead to early wear and tear. Bonus!

If you would like to learn more about orthotics, check out my book *Combat Foot Pain*, scheduled to be released by 2018.

Chapter 6: MATTRESSES AND SLEEP POSITIONS FOR NECK PAIN

FOR GOOD QUALITY SLEEP, I cannot stress the importance of having the best possible mattress. If you have neck pain, it could be due to a poor mattress! You (hopefully) sleep at least eight hours of every twenty-four hours. This is one-third of your life. If you are going to spend money on one item, it should be your mattress.

The Best Mattress That I Know Of

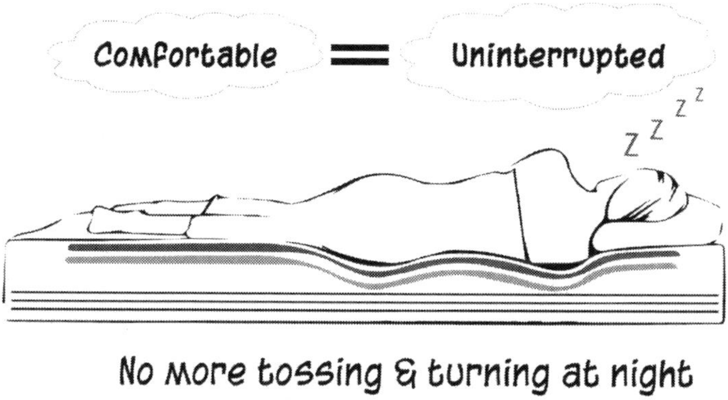

For years, I have looked for the perfect mattress. I had settled for foam mattresses, or at least mattresses topped by a foam topper. Then, finally, I came across what I consider to be *the best mattress ever.*

The Innate Sleep Orthopedic Sleep System

It took a team of engineers, guided by Dr. Rob Schroeder, a chiropractor, to create a mattress that exceeded my wildest expectations.

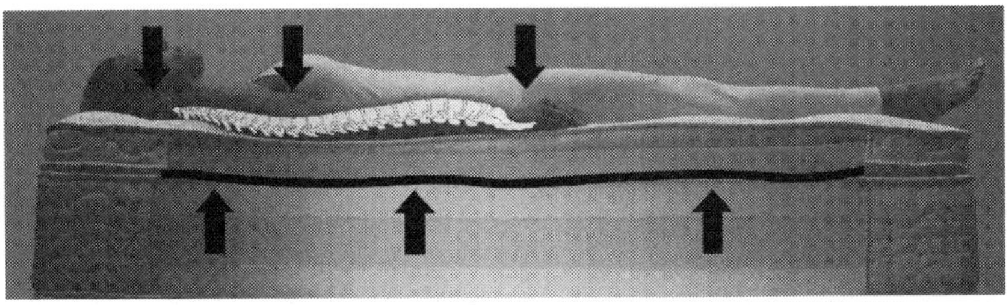

Figure 6-1: The wave action of the thin third layer of foam helps support the curves of the spine.

Unlike other foam mattresses, the Innate Sleep Orthopedic sleep system is multilayered. What separates this mattress from all other foam mattresses is its unique third layer (the dark line in Figure 6-1). This third layer is a thin yet sturdy layer of interlocking foam that bows up between two points of downward pressure.

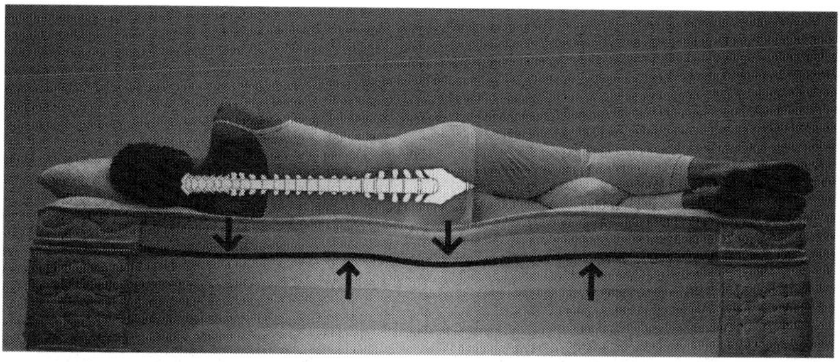

Figure 6-2: The third layer of foam creates a wave, pushing the foam up to fill in the thin areas and support the spine while keeping pressure off the thicker shoulders and hips.

Your spine is curved, and this bowing action in the mattress provides more support to these curves. It creates a wave to match the curves of your spine when you are lying on your back (Figure 6-1), or the curves of your body when you are laying on your side (Figure 6-2). It fits you whether you are large or small.

This slick design is a game changer.

Other foam mattresses are good at reducing pressure on thicker areas like your shoulders and hips, but they are not good at supporting the thinner areas like the waist and neck. This can negatively affect the low back and neck as you sink into the foam mattress (Figure 6-3).

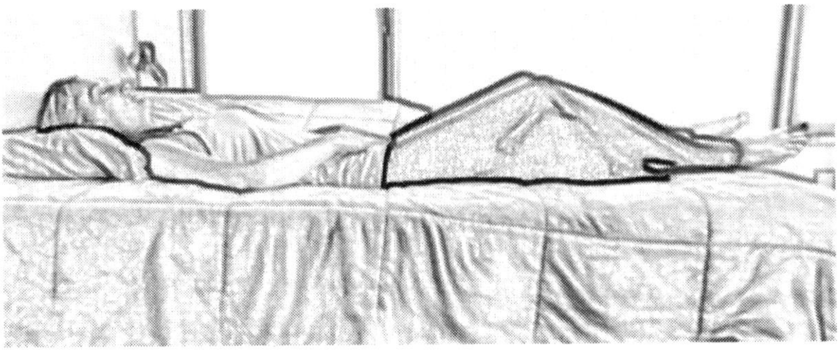

Figure 6-3: Example of lying on a foam mattress, which allows my midsection to sink too deep into the foam.

A healthy aligned spine makes an S curve. The bowing action of the third layer in the innate sleep system creates a wave that supports this curve.

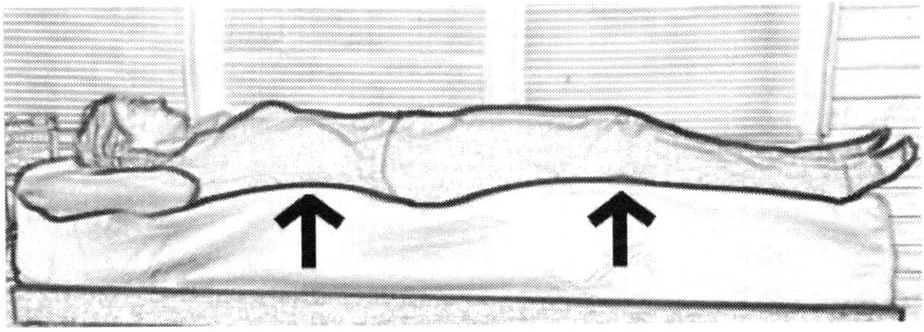

Figure 6-4: Example of the Innate Sleep System bowing upward to support the curves of the body

It is similar to how the lumbar support in the seat of a high-end car can be pumped up to support the curve of your low back while you drive. You hardly need pillows, as the mattress bows up where you need the support.

Can you see how this multilayered foam mattress is so much more than a foam mattress that just takes the pressure off the pressure points? Can you see how it is also supports the curves of your spine?

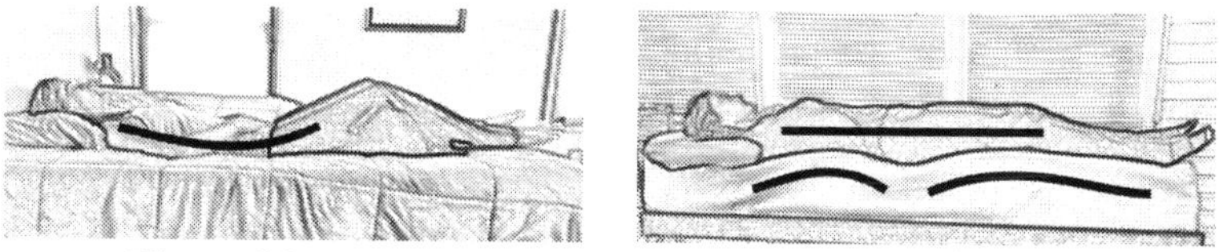

Figure 6-5: A foam mattress versus the Innate Sleep System

Bonus features of this mattress

Not only does this mattress support your spine in the best way possible, it is also earth and health friendly.

It uses botanical foam made of corn and soybean, so it doesn't give off gas like petroleum-based foam does. This was important to me because I could not sleep on my first foam mattress for months because it stank so badly.

It uses a flame-retardant cover, instead of being sprayed with toxic flame-retardant chemicals, to meet federal guidelines.

It is cheaper than other therapeutic foam mattresses. When this book was published, a king-sized bed with box springs and white-glove delivery cost $3,850.00.

Plus, the company has great customer service. It has a thirty-day no-questions-asked return policy. Plus, the company offers a fifteen-year warrantee where they will fix the mattress if the foam loses any feeling of support. You just have to pay for the material and shipping.

Foam does deteriorate over time, so the top foam layer may need to be replaced within ten years. If you choose to pay the cost of the material and shipping, you will basically have a new mattress that should last you another ten years for a few hundred dollars instead of a few thousand dollars.

The mattress is made in America (specifically Indiana).

This company has surpassed all of my expectations. It feels good to finally have a mattress I can recommend! If you would like to purchase this mattress, ask your chiropractor if they can order it for you. If not, contact me at www.drkarindc.com and I will set you up. Or you can learn more at http://innatesleep.com.

At a minimum, your mattress should be firm for support with at least an inch of foam on top to minimize pressure on your body. I recommend a separate foam topper so you can replace it every three to five years (foam loses its supportive qualities within this time). You should also flip a regular mattress every three months or so, which extends the life of the mattress.

Best Sleep Positions

The best way to sleep is on your back with contoured support. If you don't have the Innate Sleep System, you will need a contoured pillow to support your neck and a wedge pillow under your knees (refer back to Figure 6-3). When your knees are bent, your back flattens out and is better supported by the mattress.

Not only is sleeping on your back better for your neck and back, but it also keeps your face looking younger because it keeps you from rubbing the skin on your face against a pillowcase all night.

If you are a side sleeper, sleep with a thick neck pillow so your neck remains in a neutral position (Figure 6-6).

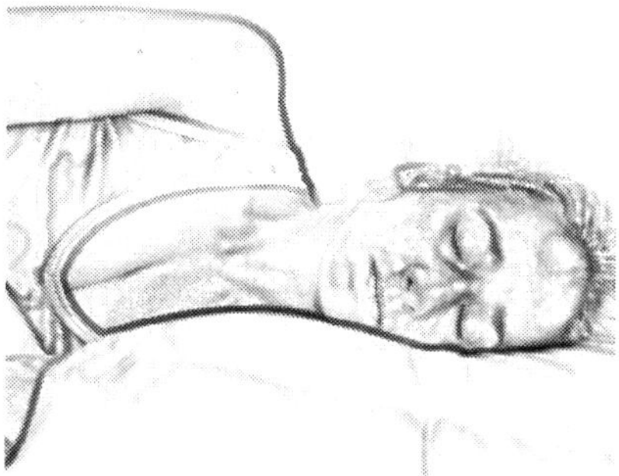

Figure 6-6: Side sleepers should use a thick pillow to support their neck.

If you sleep with your head tilted to one side, you will compress the nerves on the down side and pull on the nerves on the up side. The compression or stretching of the nerves can lead to neck pain and possibly headaches.

When sleeping on your side, you should also sleep with a pillow between your knees to keep your hips and thighs parallel to one another (helping to keep the lower half of your body in a neutral position). Otherwise, you may strain your pelvis, tailbone, hips, and/or knees as you sleep.

Choosing the Perfect Pillow

I personally use the Pillo-Pedic pillow from Foot Levelers. Because it has a soft and hard side with thick and thin edges, the Pillo-Pedic pillow is like having four pillows in one. The design makes the Pillo-Pedic great for both side and back sleepers.

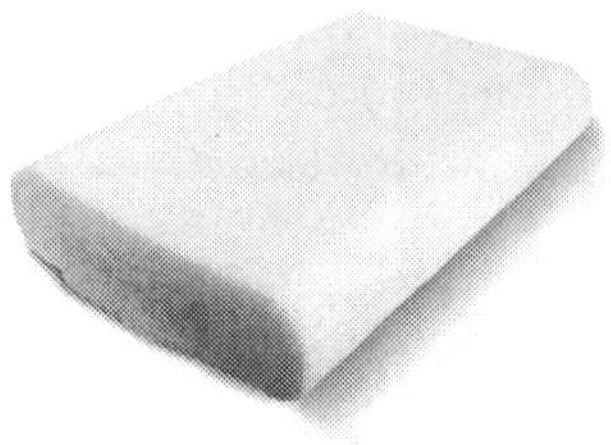

Figure 6-7: The Pillo-Pedic pillow from Foot Levelers, Inc. hard side up.

If you are a side sleeper, lay the Pillo-Pedic with the hard foam side up (Figure 6-5). When lying on your side, you don't want or need your head to sink into the pillow like you do when you are sleeping on your back.

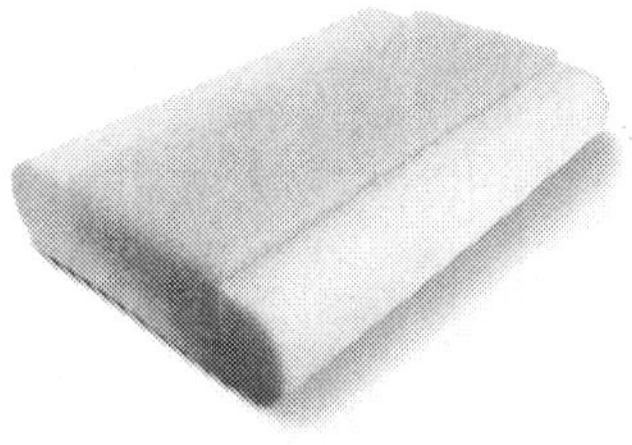

Figure 6-8: The Pillo-Pedic pillow from Foot Levelers, Inc. soft side up.

If you sleep on your back, lay it with the soft side up (Figure 6-8). This allows your head to sink into the pillow and your neck to be supported by the firmer foam edge.

The Pillo-Pedic has a thick and thin firm foam edge. Whether you lie on your back or side, place the thick edge against your shoulders if you have a long neck; use the thin edge if you have a short neck.

Foot Levelers has other pillows for your specific needs. They even offer pillows custom made from four measurements done by your healthcare provider.

To learn more, visit:
http://www.footlevelers.com/traction/index.php/pillows/exclusively-yours

Pillow advice from Dr. Rob Schroeder
President, Indy Health and Fitness
Developer of Innate Sleep Orthopedic Sleep System

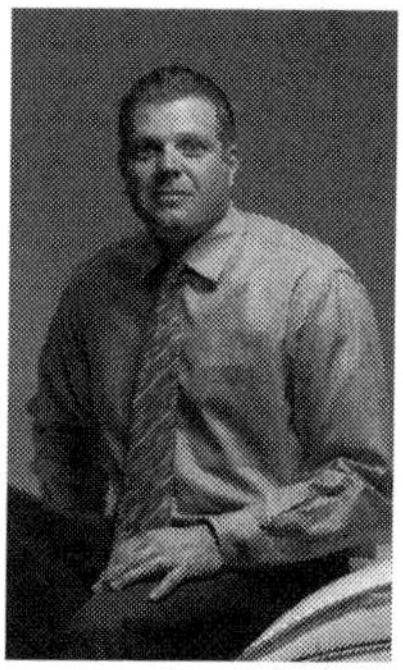

Pillows are as individual to the user as running shoes are to the marathoner. Based on the position that you sleep, the curvatures that you have in your spine, and the firmness of your mattress, your ideal pillow may be different than your neighbor's.

As a rule, I like the density of the material in the pillow to be similar to the density of the upper layers of your mattress, simply to allow the head and neck to respond to the sleep environment in the same manner as the rest of the body.

Back sleepers tend to require less height in a pillow (to avoid reversal of the lordotic curvature) with the emphasis on support being through the mid-cervical region rather than the head.

Side sleepers require more volume in their pillow to adjust to the distance between the shoulder and the neck.

Some of the contoured pillows have one end that is thin and the other that is thicker. This allows for use in both positions if the user is disciplined in positioning.

With a mattress like the Innate Sleep, where the curvatures and weight bearing are already balanced, a back sleeper needs little more than a mild roll to support the cervical curve. A side sleeper's shoulders are well absorbed by the plush layers of the mattress, which would require a thin memory foam pillow to balance the head, keeping the spine linear in this position.

The key is in the disciplined positioning of the pillow and the body to maintain ideal spinal curvatures, reduce spinal rotation, and maintain a straight spine through the long plane of the trunk. This usually takes some education, understanding, and instruction to work best.

I always suggest they discuss this with their chiropractor to be sure the positioning is ideal for the conditions that they are working on (i.e., right shoulder tendonitis patients should avoid sleeping on the right side).

Basically put…

If you wake up with neck pain, a headache, or numbness in your arms or hands, you are pinching your nerves while you sleep, and you need to change something. If you wake up with more neck pain than before you went to sleep, you probably need a new or better mattress and/or pillow. Talk to your healthcare providers and mattress stores to find someone who can help you with your specific needs.

Chapter 7: RELAXATION TECHNIQUES

STRESS IS THE NUMBER ONE CAUSE of dis-ease, which leads to disease. Having stress-induced neck pain is one example of a dis-eased state. To combat stress, you must learn to relax.

Relaxation is difficult in our culture for several reasons. First, we are all overstimulated! During our waking hours, we are bombarded with unnatural light (which messes with our sleep cycle); unnatural sounds (which are amplified by speakers and earphones blasting straight into our eardrums); potent smells (such as perfumes, colognes, and deodorants); and expectations and demands at school or work. Every one of these is a potential trigger for stress, leading to neck pain and headaches.

So how can we relax despite all of this?

Breathe

You have a huge diaphragm muscle that is designed to move with every breath. On average, you take 960 breaths an hour, 23,040 breaths a day, and 8,409,600 breaths a year. When you are stressed, you tend to breathe more shallowly with your accessory breathing muscles (like the anterior scalenes). These muscles were not designed to move with every breath.

Your upper lungs are smaller than your lower lungs. If you only breathe into your upper lungs, you deprive yourself of the full amount of oxygen your body requires. Oxygen deprivation is another stressor that can lead to muscle tension and neck pain.

This is why deep breathing is not only calming, but healthier. As you breathe fully into your lungs, you improve the oxygen and carbon dioxide transfer, which supplies your body with much-needed oxygen and rids it of toxic carbon dioxide.

Try taking a moment to focus on breathing out twice as long as you breathe in. If you can maintain this breathing pattern for more than five minutes, you should feel the tension in your body melting away. This technique is used in meditation practices. An added benefit of this breathing technique is that it increases the oxygen in your blood, which may help alleviate your neck pain.

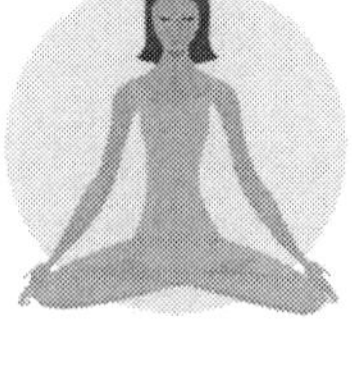

Tense and Relax

If you are not relaxing with a breathing technique alone, focus on relaxing different body parts. Most people find it is easier to tense (or contract) a muscle than to relax it, so to relax your whole body, try this tense-and-relax exercise.

I recommend doing this laying on your back so you can work toward relaxing all of your muscles. You can also do this seated or standing, but that limits how many muscles you can truly relax because some will have to remain contracted to hold you upright. It may be more comfortable to lay on your back with a pillow under your knees (remember Figure 6-2).

Start by tensing your toes and then relaxing them. Then move your attention up to the calf muscles. Tense them, then relax them. Move up to your thigh muscles. Contract the front thigh muscles, then relax them. Contract the posterior thigh muscles, then relax them. Move up to the pelvic bowl, do a kegel, and then relax. Move to the lower back, and contract and relax the lower back muscles.

Continue up the back, contracting and relaxing as you go. Move down the arms, all the way to the fingertips, contracting and relaxing the muscles as you go. Return to the shoulders, and contract and relax the individual muscles. Move up the neck, contract the muscles in the back of the neck, and relax. Contract the muscles in the front of the neck, and relax.

Contract and relax your facial muscles (smile and frown). Contract and relax your tongue (curl your tongue, stick it out), your jaw muscles (open and close your mouth), and your eye muscles (look up, down, right, and left). By the time you reach your forehead (raise and lower your eyebrows), your whole body should be relaxed.

The added benefit of this relaxation technique is that if your neck pain is from the tension in your neck, jaw, upper back, or any other muscle, contracting and relaxing your muscles will help alleviate your neck pain.

If you have a hard time relaxing with these techniques, you may want to try R.E.S.T., also known as floatation therapy and sensory deprivation therapy. I describe this in the next chapter.

Chapter 8: R.E.S.T.: RESTRICTED ENVIRONMENTAL STIMULATION THERAPY

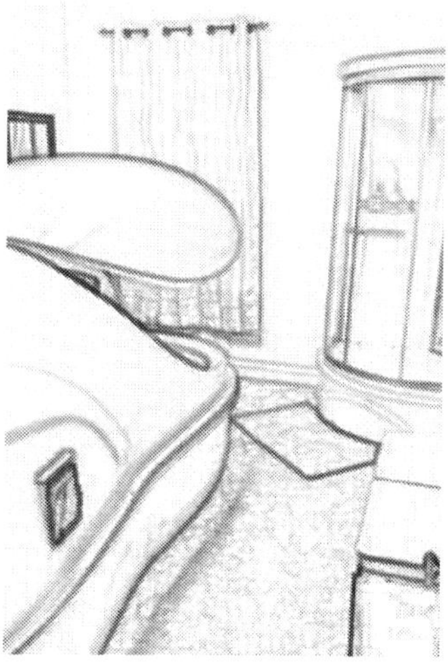

Figure 8-1: Dr. Karin's floatation pod.

RESTRICTED Environmental Stimulation Therapy, also known as sensory deprivation therapy, is a great therapy to use to relax and de-stress. I got one mainly for myself, as stress is a cause of dis-ease, which leads to disease. Being a working mother, I have several stressors in my life.

I work hard and play hard, and floating is a great way to relieve muscle soreness and to promote relaxation. It was a bonus that I was able to provide my patients with a therapy that is becoming more common in America, especially because it helps a large array of ailments.

What Is a Floatation Pod?

A floatation pod (Figure 8-1) is a huge capsule that is sealed from light and sound to provide R.E.S.T. (Restricted Environmental Stimulation Therapy). It has 100 gallons of water saturated with 900 pounds of Epsom salts.

Many people take Epsom salt baths to help ease their muscle aches and pains. Can you imagine what 900 pounds of Epsom salts will do for your muscles?

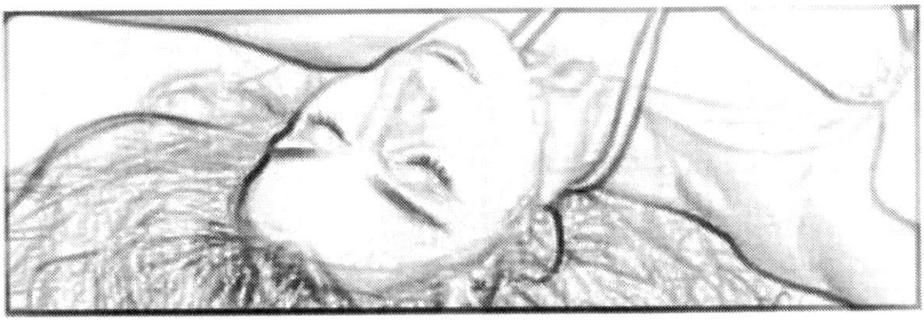

Not only that, but due to the concentration of the salt, you float effortlessly on the water. The body is less dense than this solution of water, so it floats like a cork does in water. This allows your muscles to relax from the inside out.

Once fully relaxed, you feel the space between your bones elongate and the pressure on nerves decrease. Your blood flow and lymph drainage also increase. The body is in a state that allows it to heal on a deeper level. Many people report that not only does their pain decrease, but a sense of euphoria comes over them.

The Benefits of Floating

I got interested in floatation therapy because it is the most effective treatment for helping people relax, making it an effective treatment for all kinds of ailments, including neck tension and pain. The sensory deprivation also allows the brain to calm down, heal, and replenish.

In a floatation pod, breathing deepens, the heart rate slows, blood pressure decreases, stress hormone levels decrease, and you experience a sense of euphoria and well-being. You become less sensitive to pain once you reach this state.

Brain Waves

There are different brain waves detectible by instrumentation (Figure 8-2):

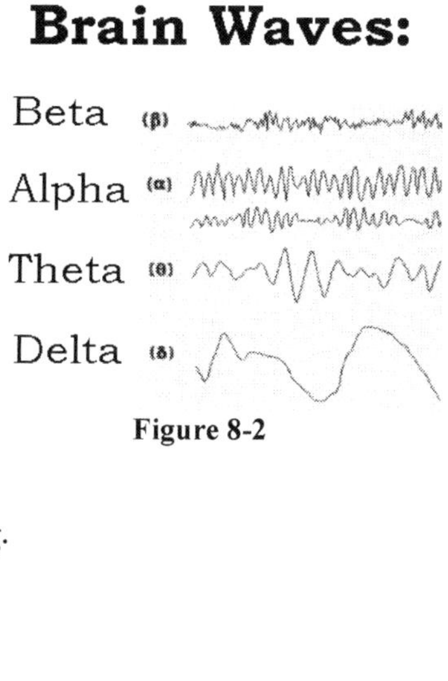

Figure 8-2

1. The **beta brain wave** is associated with being aware, understanding, engaging, and actively thinking.

2. The **delta brain wave**, in contrast, is associated with sleeping.

3. The **alpha brain wave** is between the two; it represents a daydream-like state.

4. Then there is the elusive **theta brain wave** state. It is the state when the brain is "being"—when the person is not asleep, but not actively thinking or daydreaming either. This is the state that master gurus of meditation can attain despite external stimulation. This state is the most deficient in our culture.

Why Are Most of Us Deficient in Theta Waves?

Remember, we are all overstimulated! Most of us are overstimulated until the moment we finally crash from our awake (beta/alpha) state to our sleep (delta) state, skipping the healing theta brain wave state. Worse yet, we are rudely awakened by an irritating alarm sound, quickly transitioning from our delta (sleep) to beta (awake) state, again skipping the much-needed healing theta brain wave state.

Feeling myself theta deprived, I bought a floatation pod to help me get into a theta brain wave state, to relax, and to help me tap into the brain's ability to facilitate healing.

Stress is the number one cause of disease (what I like to call *dis-ease,* because the body's state of unease makes it vulnerable to disease). So I value any way to decrease stress: meditating, exercising, laughing with friends, and now floatation therapy.

How Floatation Helps Neck Pain

Remember, one of the causes of neck pain is stress. Stress can cause sleep deprivation. Sometimes neck pain can affect sleep. This can lead to a vicious cycle. You can break this cycle by resting in a float pod.

One hour of floating is like several hours of sleeping. People who suffer from insomnia benefit from floating because they often can sleep in the pod. Many also report that they fall asleep more easily afterward and their quality of sleep improves.

Tension is another cause of neck pain. Floating allows the muscles to relax because your body does not have work against gravity to keep you upright. The Epsom salt also aids in muscle relaxation.

Many of my patients report a significant reduction of their neck pain with floatation. The only variables are the duration and degree of the relief.

If you want to learn more about floatation therapy, check out the largest floatation center in the United States, located in Portland, Oregon: http://floathq.com/

Chapter 9: FLOOR STRETCHES AND EXERCISES FOR NECK HEALTH

AFTER BEING INVOLVED in a car crash, I could barely move. My neck pain was too acute and swollen to manipulate, so stretching my neck and doing passive modalities like electrical muscle stimulation, massage, and kinesio taping my neck was my only option.

I cannot stress enough that if you have neck pain, it is imperative that you stretch your tight muscles and strengthen your loose muscles. When your muscles aren't too tight and aren't too loose, you will hold the beneficial effects of your treatments longer and be less vulnerable to injury. Research supports that home exercise is more effective than taking medicine.[1]

In this chapter, I share some of the floor exercises and stretches I used to loosen up my neck and back. I was determined to go from having a stiff, almost immobilized spine to one that could move enough to do my activities of daily living.

---

[1] Bronfort et al., "Spinal Manipulation," *Annals of Internal Medicine.*

Stretching the Neck

To loosen up your neck, turn your head from side to side and then tilt your head left and right.

To work on the extension of your spine, lie on your stomach, face down on the mat, with your hands palm up at your sides. With your nose and chin on the mat, carefully lift your head a off the mat using your back muscles (Figures 9-1 and 9-2).

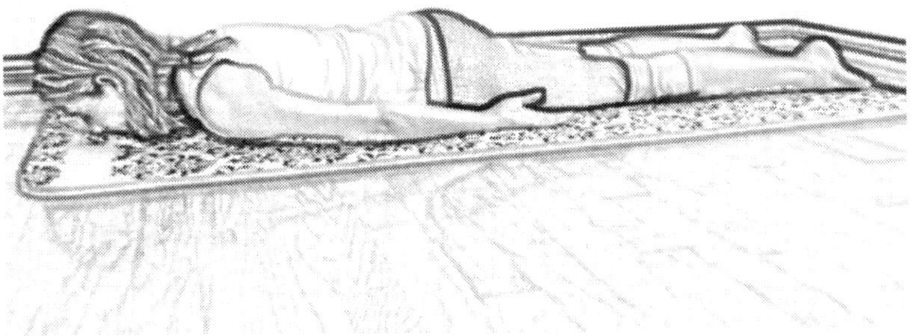

Figure 9-1: Lying prone (face down) on the mat, rest your chin on the mat.

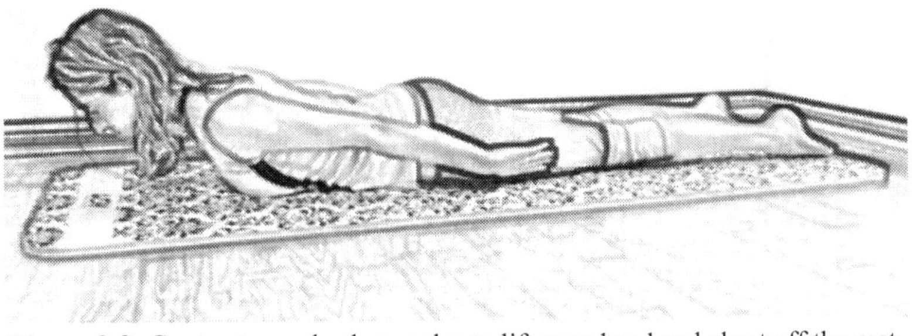

Figure 9-2: Contract your back muscles to lift your head and chest off the mat.

Then slowly lower your head, resting your head on the mat turned to the right as far as possible (Figure 9-3). You may not be able to turn your head all the way to the right, and that is fine. Just turn your head as far as you comfortably can. After going through this routine a couple of times, your neck should loosen up. Your range of motion will improve a little bit with each repetition.

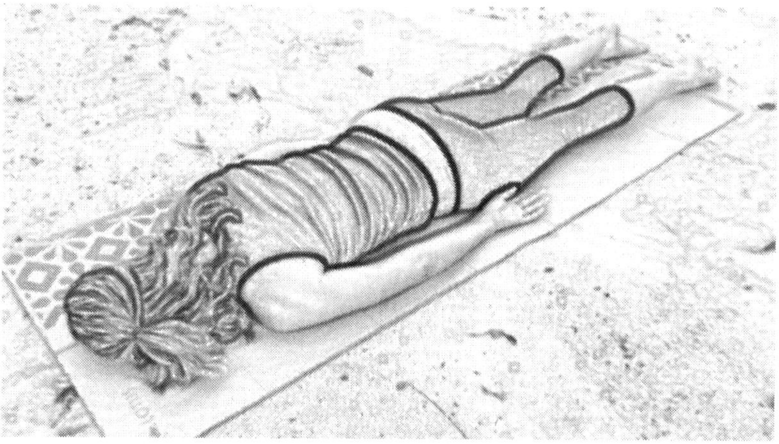

Figure 9-3: Strong stretch for the neck to the right.

Once your neck relaxes, bring your head back to center, and raise your head slightly again (Figure 9-4). If it feels like you are straining, back off. If not, lift it higher. You can place your arms in front of you to support your upper body if you need to.

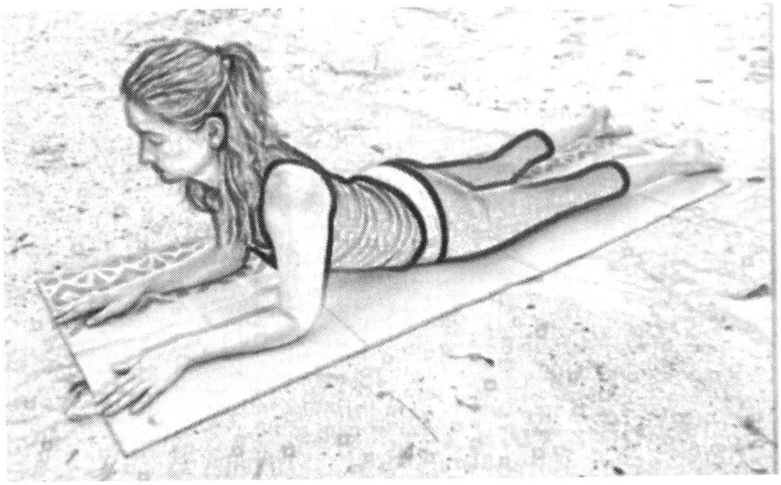

Figure 9-4: Passive back bend.

Then lower your head back onto the mat with your head turned to the left (Figure 9-5). Relax, allowing your muscles to elongate.

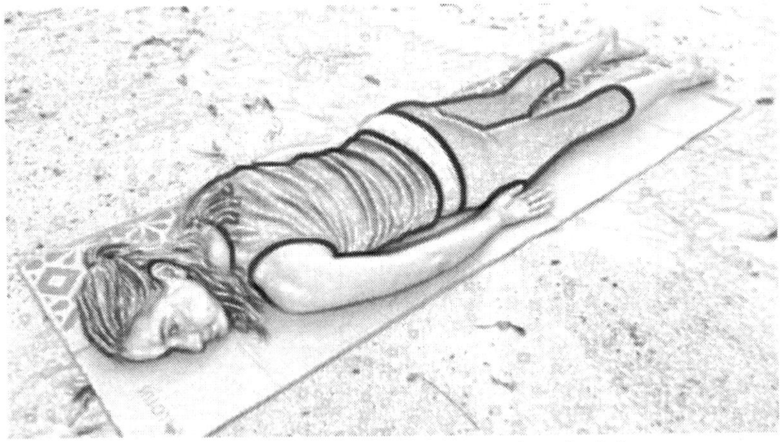

Figure 9-5: Strong stretch for the neck to the left.

Then bring your head to the center and repeat the series of moves. Go a little bit higher each time without straining yourself. Repeat three times.

When your neck does not feel any strain when you lift it off the mat, bring your hands under your shoulders, squeeze them muscles between your shoulder blades to lift your hands as you raise your head (to strengthen your back muscles and work on your back extension; Figure 9-6).

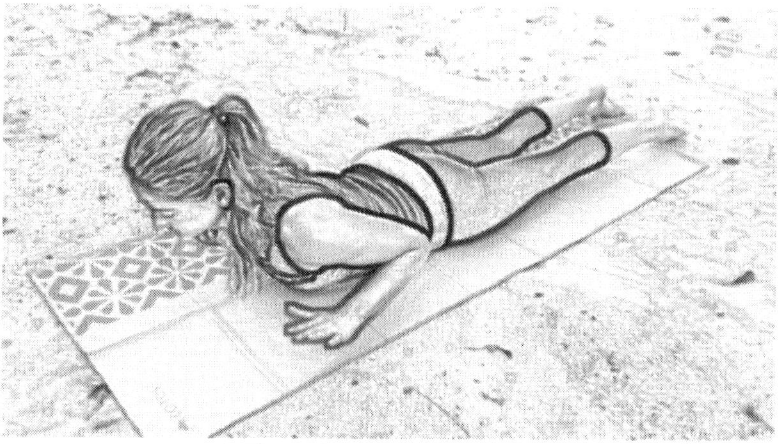

Figure 9-6: Active back bend.

Again, move very slowly and concentrate on your breath (breathing in with lifting, breathing out with lowering) and form (keeping your shoulder blades down and engaged).

Stretching the Back

Get on your hands and knees to do cat and cow poses (Figure 9-7), breathing in with cow and breathing out with cat. This is a great way to loosen up your mid-back. Repeat the sequence three to five times.

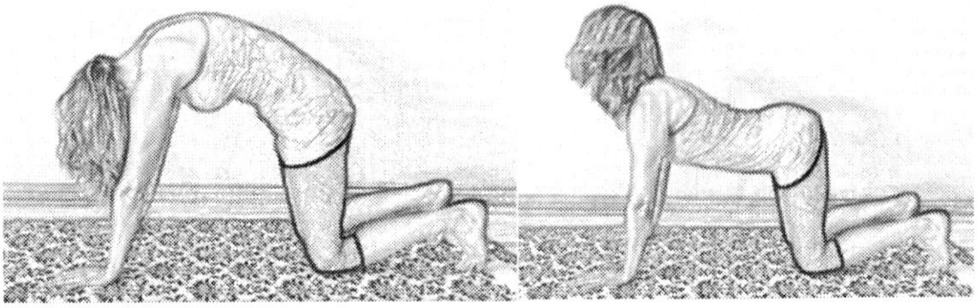

Figure 9-7: Cat and cow pose.

Then roll onto your back to do some additional back stretches, which can help ease your neck pain.

Start with the basic passive back bend. You only need two items to make this stretch effective. The first is a soft, flat surface. Figure 9-8 shows me using a mat because my floors are hardwood. A mat provides some cushioning between your body and the floor. You could also simply lie on the carpet or a rug; just make sure you have enough cushion for your back to feel comfortable.

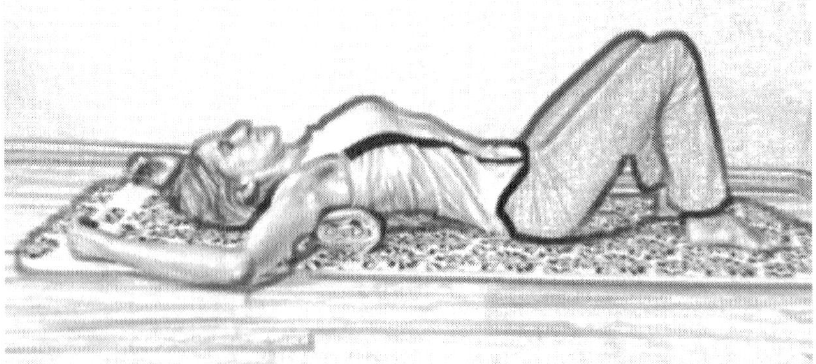

Figure 9-8: Passive back bend with a rolled-up towel.

The second item you need is a large towel. Roll the bath towel into a tube and place it perpendicularly on the mat or floor.

Lay down so the towel is behind your back at the level of your shoulder blades (Figure 9-8). You can place your arms along your sides. For a deeper stretch, raise your arms above your head along the mat. This helps passively extend your back.

If you need a deeper stretch, use a foam roller instead of a rolled-up towel (Figure 9-9).

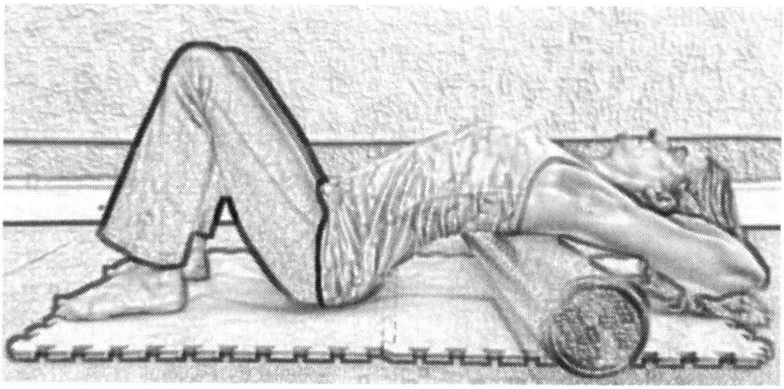

Figure 9-9: Strong passive back bend.

Lay in this position as long as is comfortable, but no longer than five minutes at one time. If you stay in this position too long, you may elongate your ligaments to a point that you may be vulnerable to moving your spine incorrectly, which could result in you tweaking your back.

Extending your spine this way helps counteract reaching and/or slouching all day. If you don't take the time to work on the extension of your mid-back, you will become more rigid in your forward bend, which strains your neck over time.

Stronger Passive Back Bends

You can also use an exercise ball to do a passive back bend. I advise people to sit on an exercise ball for twenty minutes every hour or so, whether you're at home or at the office. Using an exercise ball is a great way to move while you sit, and then you can use it to do passive back bends throughout the day.

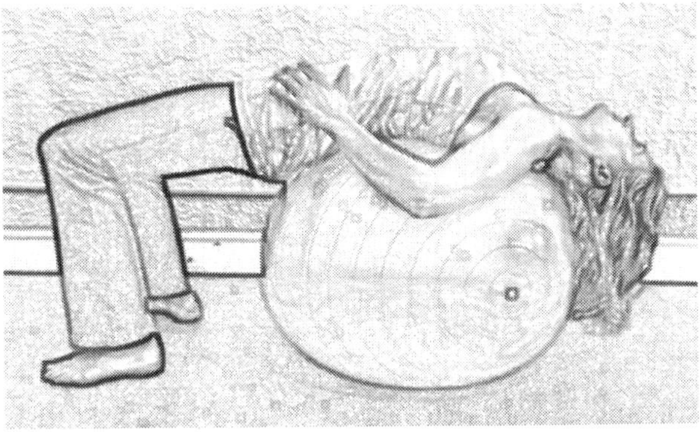

Figure 9-10: Passive back bend over an exercise ball.

To do a passive back bend on an exercise ball, simply sit on the floor holding the ball behind you. Then move up the ball as it rolls under you until you are arching your back over the ball as far as you comfortably can (Figure 9-10).

Frequency is more important than intensity or duration with this stretch. You can stay in this position for a few slow breaths and then repeat it throughout the day. This is why it's nice to have an exercise ball at work; you can sit on it for twenty minutes, stretch on it, stand for twenty minutes, stretch on the ball, and sit again.

As you become more flexible and get more comfortable moving on the ball, you can do a full back bend on the exercise ball.

This requires you to roll back on the ball and then reach your arms and hands over your head to brace yourself on the floor (Figure 9-11). This is a more comprehensive stretch in that it works your arm, back, thigh, calf, and feet muscles, not to mention your abs.

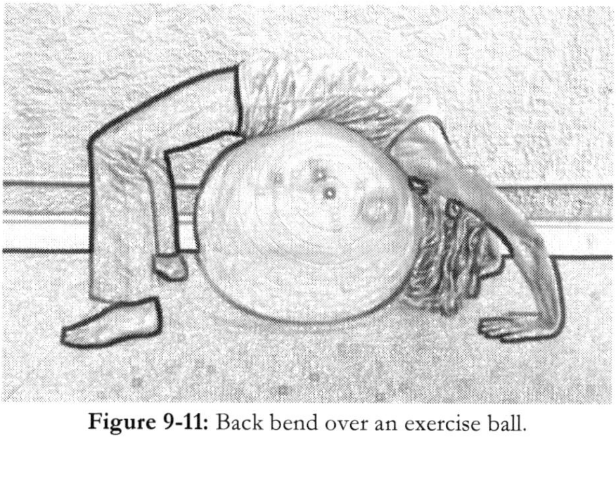

Figure 9-11: Back bend over an exercise ball.

Wheel Pose

After you are comfortable doing back bends on the exercise ball, you can work toward doing the wheel pose, which is shown in Figure 9-12.

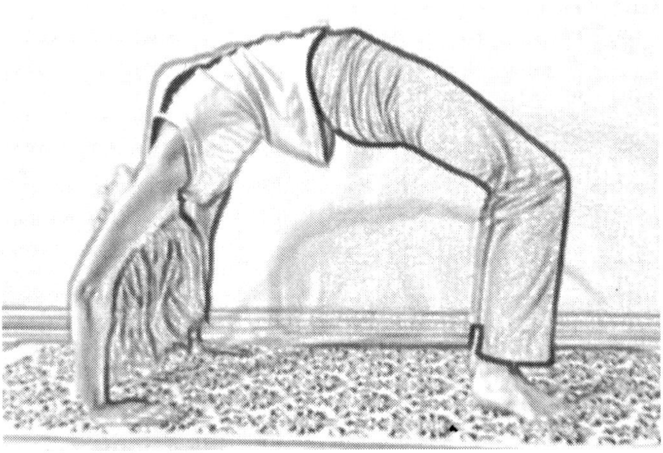

Figure 9-12: Wheel pose.

It took me over a year of daily stretching and strengthening to get back to doing the wheel pose after my crash. If you have no experience with the wheel pose, see a yoga instructor for the best way to enter this pose. This pose is as hard as it looks, and if you don't understand the proper way to get into and out of it, you could injure yourself. It's best to master the other back bends in this chapter before attempting the wheel pose.

Mountain Pose

The mountain pose is a standing stretch. Check your plumb line, making sure your ears are over your shoulders, your shoulders are over your hips, and your hips are over your knees and ankles (Figure 9-13).

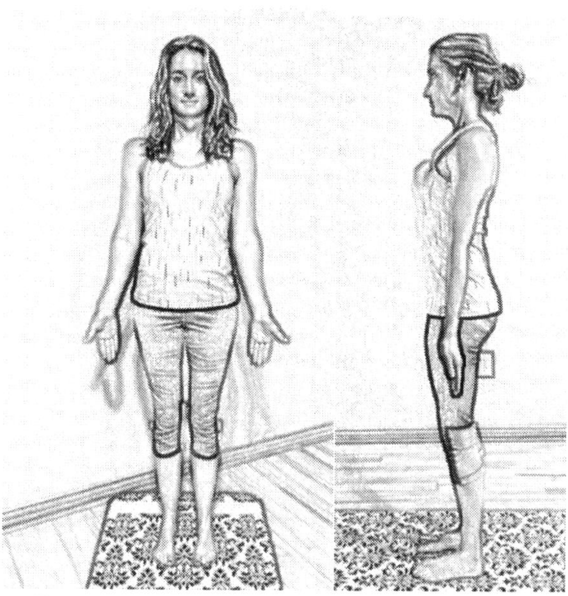

Figure 9-13: Mountain pose from the front and side.

Plant your feet onto the mat. Make sure your toes are spread apart and you can feel your heels pressing evenly into the ground. The base of your big and little toes should bear equal weight. This triangular pattern of weight bearing on the feet is important for stabilization of the pose. This pose strengthens the muscles that are involved with holding a healthy posture, which is imperative for a healthy neck.

Working toward Forward Bends

A human head weighs an average of 10 pounds. That's a lot of weight for your neck to support day in and day out. Just think how nice it would feel to be able to hang your head upside down and let gravity pull your head and neck in the opposite direction. Forward bends allow you to achieve this. But most people have to work up to the ultimate forward bend, where you look like you're bent in half at the waist.

One of the things I like about forward bends is that they work so many other muscles at the same time. So, while you're working to loosen your neck muscles, you're stretching other muscles.

Begin a forward bend by bending forward at the waist (Figure 9-14). Make sure you lead with your chest and not your head. If you strain to reach farther, you may harm your back versus stretching your muscles.

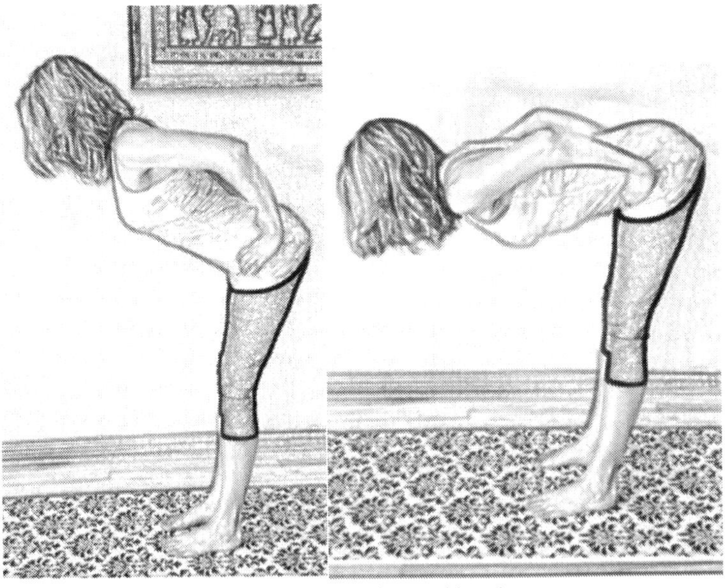

Figure 9-14: A forward bend.

Keep your back in a neutral position as you hinge forward at the waist. You may not go as far as I am in Figure 9-14, but if you are feeling a stretch, you are improving the mobility of the muscles you are feeling the stretch in. So as you hinge forward, pay attention to where you are feeling the stretch. If you are feeling a stretch in your hamstrings (the back of your thighs), then great! You are stretching your hamstrings!

If you are feeling a strain in your back, you are *straining* your back. Stop! Come back up and try again.

Aim to reach your hands to the mat (Figure 9-15), keeping your back as neutral as possible, to keep the stretch in your hamstrings.

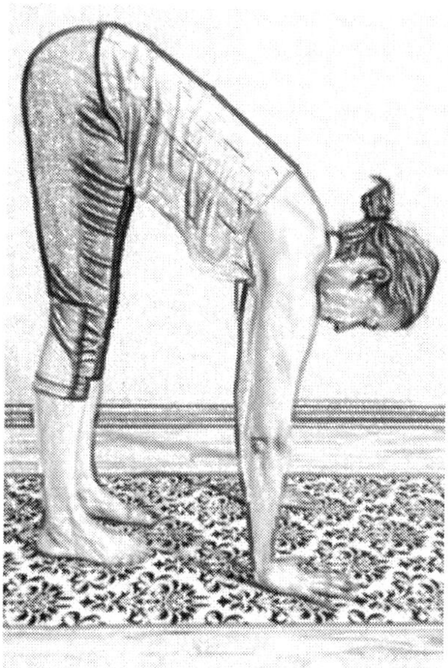

Figure 9-15: Forward bend with hands to mat, keeping the back flat.

It may take months or even years before you can press your palms to the mat, but your range of motion will improve in the process. Maybe you can work toward getting your hands to the floor or your nose to your knees (Figure 9-16). Whatever your goal, as long as you improve or maintain over time, you are a success!

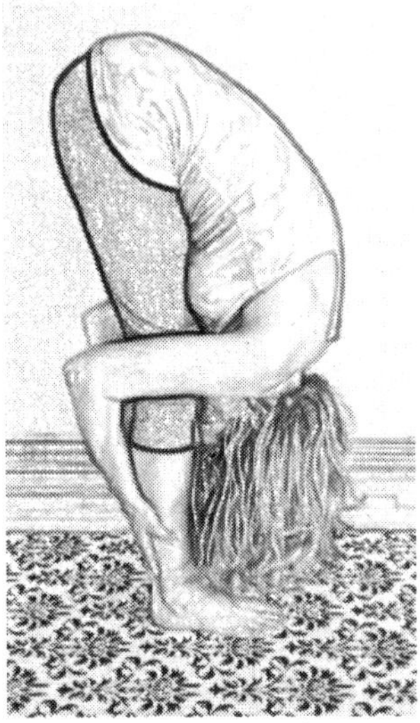

Figure 9-16: The ultimate forward bend.

Forward bends are a great way to traction your neck with the weight of your head.

Being Aware of Your Body in Space

If your neck pain is due to an injury, you may need to work on your *proprioception* (the awareness of your body in space without using your vision or inner ears). The body is not quite the same after an injury, no matter how minor, so I always have my patients check their proprioception. Proprioception allows you to correct off-balance movements and prevent falls caused by imbalance. Jarring actions of even catching yourself from falling can re-exacerbate neck pain. Strengthening your awareness of where your body is in space will make you less vulnerable to any type of re-injury.

You can test your proprioception by standing on one foot and closing your eyes (Figure 9-17). With your eyes closed, you can't rely on your vision to tell you where you are in space. Because you are not moving, your inner ears can't help you either. You are relying solely on your proprioception.

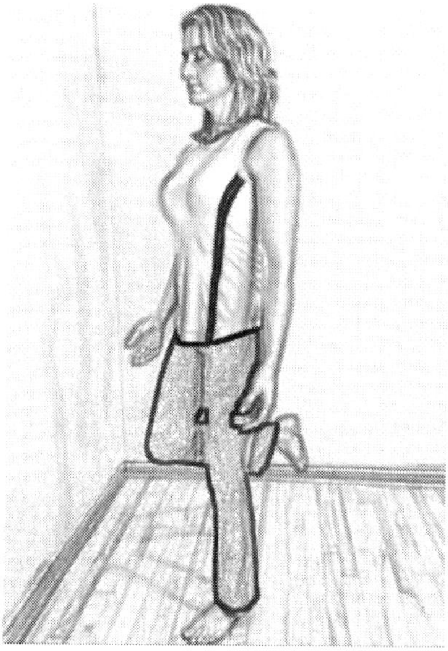

Figure 9-17: Testing my proprioception.

If any bone in your body is misaligned, you will have a difficult time standing on one foot with your eyes closed because your brain automatically sends signals to your muscles to make minor adjustments to keep your body upright. If your body isn't aligned as your brain expects, the muscle corrections will actually be incorrect and you will start wobbling.

If you can't stand on one leg with your eyes closed for more than thirty seconds (three minutes on a wobble board if you are in sports), then you are more prone to injuries because you are visually dependent for your balance. If you get visually distracted for a short period of time, you will likely misjudge where you are in space and potentially get hurt (misplace your foot and roll your ankle for example).

Proprioception Exercise

Most people lose their balance as they age. I attribute this to the fact that many people do not exercise their balance. How often do you stand on one foot with your eyes closed? If you don't use it, you lose it.

In addition to relying on your vision to tell you where you are in your surroundings, you have mechanisms in your inner ears that tell your brain how you are moving. Nerve fibers throughout your body give your brain even more input as to where you are in space.

To exercise your body's proprioception, you need to remove two indicators of your body's position: sight and detection of movement by your inner ears. You can do this by closing your eyes (to remove the visual reference) and standing still on one leg (without movement, your inner ears aren't much assistance). You should do this by a wall or with your hands hovering over a counter so you can prevent yourself from falling if you start to wobble too much (Figure 9-18).

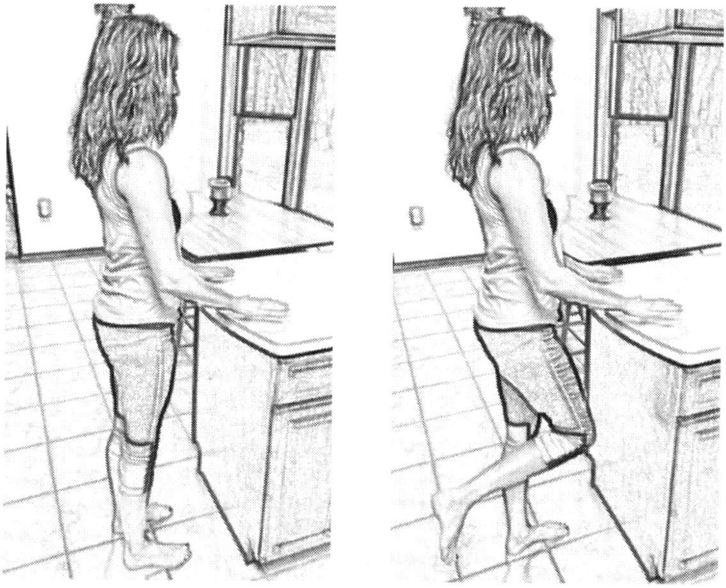

Figure 9-18: Working on proprioception while hovering my hands over a counter, eyes closed, and standing with one foot off the floor.

You should be able to do this for at least thirty seconds per leg (three minutes if you are an athlete). If you cannot, then you are vulnerable to injury if you get visually distracted and misstep. Good proprioception allows you to catch yourself from falling, making you less likely to twist an ankle (or, when you're elderly, break a bone). If you don't practice your proprioception, you are more likely to fall, resulting in injury.

Everyone should do this exercise every day. People sit too much, often with poor posture. If you don't fight the effects of sitting, you become more bent and stiff with time. Your brain doesn't notice this slow process, and when you reach that tipping point, you start misjudging where you are in space to such a degree that you become clumsy. I have had patients who started having multiple falls in situations where they shouldn't, for example, when going from carpets to hard flooring. Once they worked on their proprioception, they didn't fall as often (if at all).

Once you can comfortably stand on one leg with your eyes closed for thirty seconds, you may be able to do this exercise next to a wall, making it easier to do throughout the day.

Chapter 10: SEATED STRETCHES TO HELP RELIEVE NECK AND ARM PAIN

MOST NECK PAIN involves tight posterior neck muscles, weak muscles between the shoulder blades, and tight pectoral (chest) muscles. This chapter shows you how to stretch the posterior neck muscles and tight pectoral muscles.

These stretches are good for alleviating neck pain, headaches, and pain that radiates down the arms, all of which can be a result of poor posture, poor work ergonomics, injury, and/or degeneration over time.

Unless otherwise noted, you can do these stretches either sitting or standing. If you sit at a desk all day, I encourage you to stand up when stretching.

Most of these stretches are in my *Top Seven Ways to Combat the Effects of Sitting* book. If you have read this book, you can skip this chapter (unless you need a refresher on the exercises).

As always, confirm with your health provider that these stretches are safe and appropriate for you.

Neck Rotation

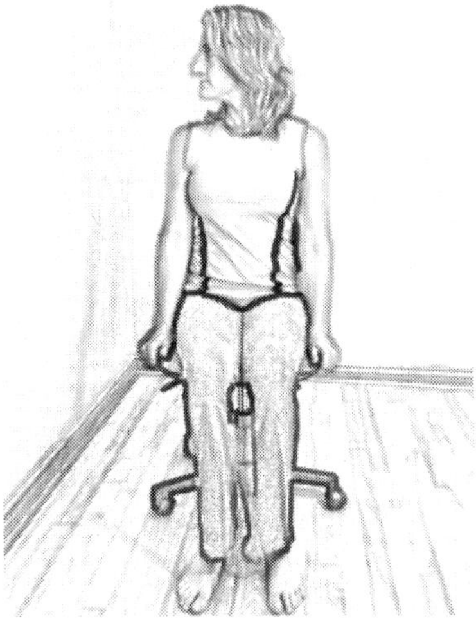

Figure 10-1

Simply turning your neck left and right will stretch the muscles of your neck and upper back (Figure 10-1). Turn your head to the right until it's in line with your shoulder. Hold the position. Then repeat on the left. Keep your shoulders down and away from your ears during this stretch.

These movements don't take long and are easy to sneak in throughout the day. Even during a meeting, you can take a moment to look far to the right and left.

Neck Flexion

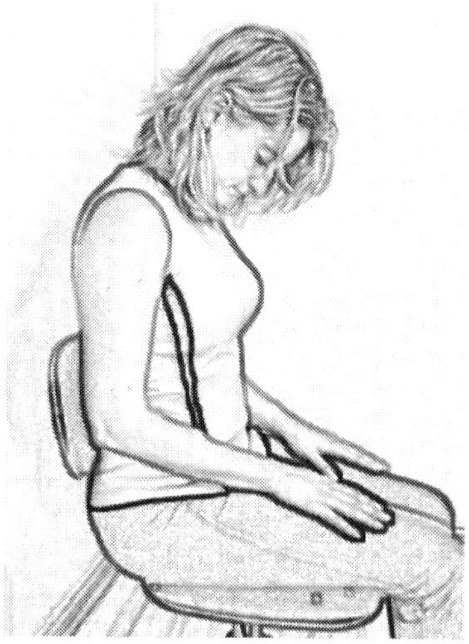

Figure 10-2

To perform the neck flexion, look down and tuck your chin in to stretch the upper back muscles (Figure 10-2). People tend to sit with their chins jutted out, which elongates and weakens the muscles in the front of the neck. Tucking your chin in adds to the stretch in the muscles in the back of the neck and strengthens the muscles in the front of your neck.

Neck Lateral Flexion

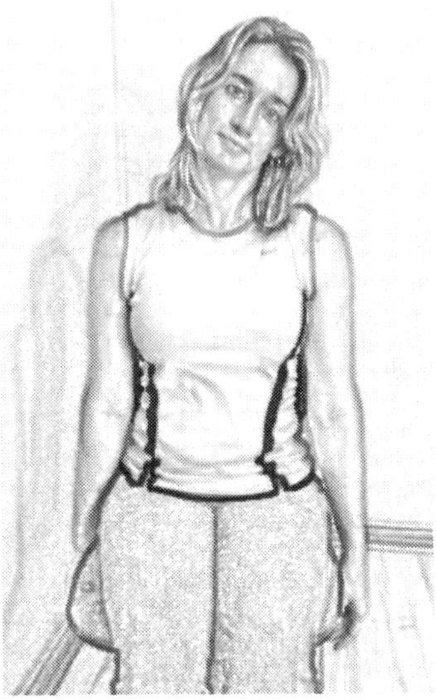

Figure 10-3

When you perform the neck lateral flexion stretch, you stretch the muscles in the sides of your neck. To do this stretch, hold your chair seat with your right hand to anchor your right shoulder down as you tilt your head to the left (Figure 10-3). You can lean your head slightly forward and back to stretch different muscle in the side of your neck. Hold each position for at least three breaths, and then repeat on the other side to stretch the left lateral neck muscles.

If you are standing, hold your right wrist with your left hand to anchor your right shoulder down as you tilt your head to the left. Again, you can lean your head slightly forward and back to stretch different muscles in your neck. Hold each position for at least three breaths. Repeat on the other side.

You can deepen this stretch even further. When stretching the right side of your neck, stretch your right hand to point your fingertips down and slightly out. Then. using your left hand, reach across the top of your head and gently press on the right side of your head to slightly extend the stretch. Be careful not to press too hard; the goal is to stretch your neck, not strain it. Keep your shoulders down and away from your ears. Repeat on the other side.

Shoulder Rolls

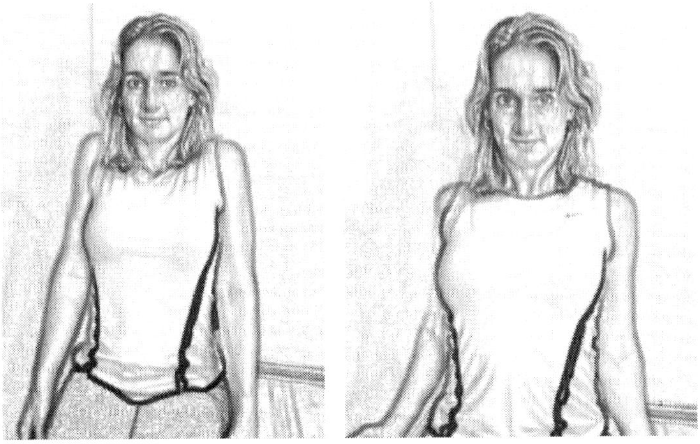

Figure 10-4

To loosen your upper back and shoulder muscles, raise your shoulders to your ears and then roll them as far back as you can and as far down away from your ears as you can (Figure 10-4). Move them forward and back up to complete the circle. Slowly repeat this rotation five times.

Breathe in as you raise your shoulders, and breathe out as you roll them back and down. This allows you to combine stretching with a calming breath, which helps calm the mind (an important activity to do throughout a stressful work day). Remember, stress is the cause of all dis-ease that leads to disease. So find ways like this to relax, rejuvenate, and heal throughout the day.

Arms Over Head Stretch

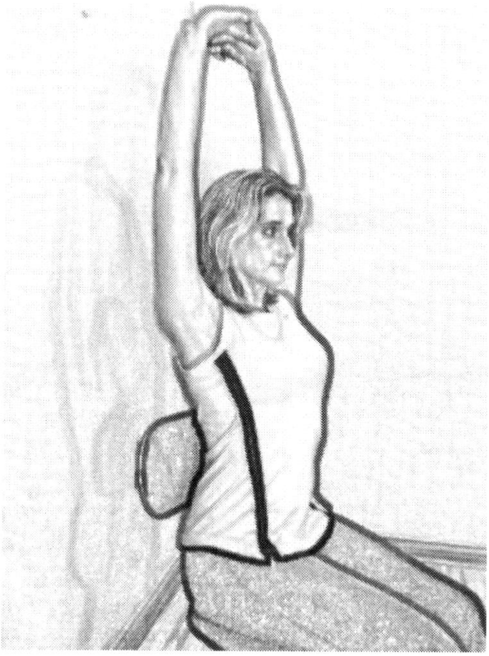

Figure 10-5

When you stretch your arms over your head, you work the muscles in your back and shoulders. To do this stretch, interlace your fingers and stretch your arms straight up over your head with your palms turned up (Figure 10-5). Keep your shoulders away from your ears and your elbows straight. Hold your arms above your head and breathe five slow breaths.

If you do this stretch while standing, be careful not to hyperextend your lower back by sticking your buttocks out too far. Keep space in your low back as you lift your arms up and back.

External Shoulder Rotation

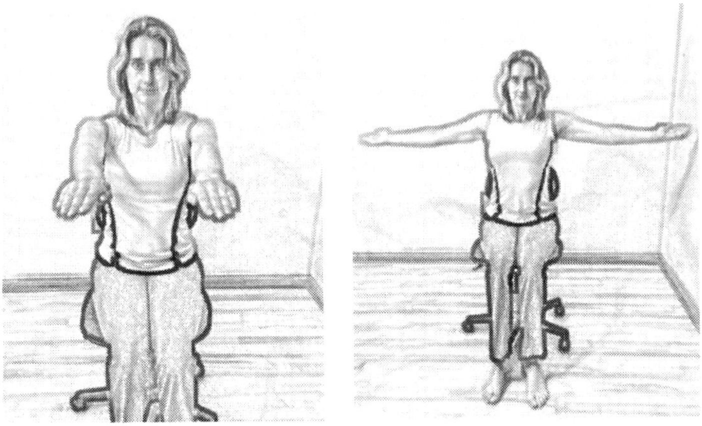

Figure 10-6

To do the external shoulder rotation, stretch your arms out in front of you, palms down (Figure 10-6). Then extend your arms to the sides, moving horizontally, while rotating your palms upward. Be sure to engage the muscles between your shoulder blades as you bring your arms out.

Reverse the movement, slowly bringing your arms forward and rotating your palms down. Repeat the stretch a few times. This warms up the shoulders and works on external rotation (a movement we don't do naturally while working at a computer).

Arm Raise

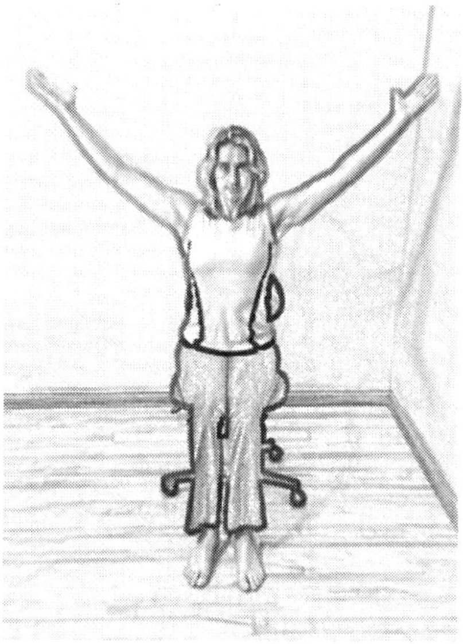

Figure 10-7

When you sit (often hunched over) at your computer for hours, your arms and palm down the whole time unless you mindfully do a stretch like this. To do the arm raise, bring your arms up, palms up, to form a V, and squeeze your shoulders back and down (Figure 10-7). Slowly lower them back to your sides and repeat a few times. Do this stretch frequently to offset the effects of long-term keyboard use.

This stretch helps old blood and lymph drain out of the upper extremities. When you lower your arms, nutrient-filled blood replenishes them (helping you heal from conditions like carpal tunnel or tendonitis). I like to do this stretch at least once an hour while at a computer. It stretches your lateral side muscles (latissimus dorsi) and strengthens your rhomboid muscles.

Hands Behind Head Neck Traction

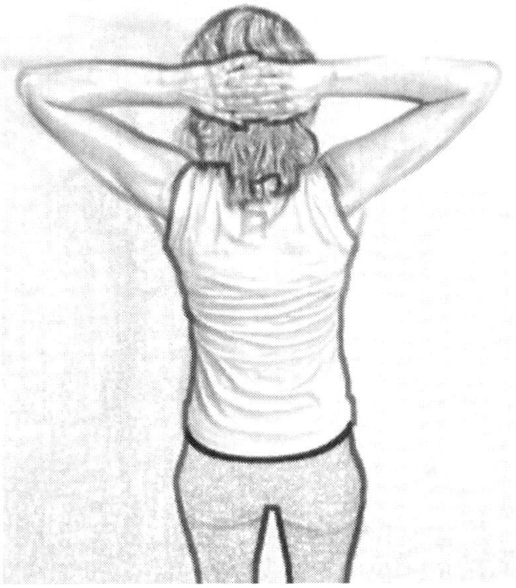

Figure 10-8

All day long, your arms are down in front of you. This stretch involves doing the opposite of what you do all day. Interlace your fingers behind your head (Figure 10-8). Tuck your chin in, press your head back into your hands, and squeeze your shoulder blades together. Hold this for five breaths. This stretch stretches the back of your neck and the front of your chest while strengthening the mid-back muscles.

This stretch can be done while seated or standing. If you are standing, be careful not to arch your back too much into extension (you want the mid-back to arch, not the lower back to compress).

Pectoral Stretch

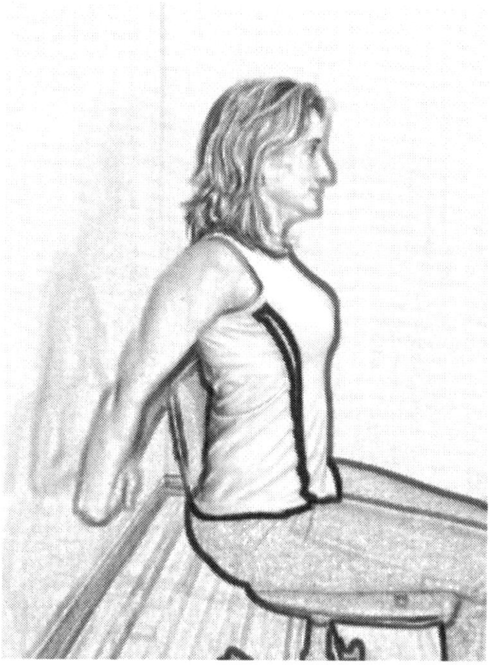

Figure 10-9

The pectorals are the muscles in the upper chest. To stretch these muscles, place your hands behind your back and interlace your fingers (Figure 10-9). Straighten your elbows and lift your hands away from your buttocks (squeezing your shoulder blades together). In addition to stretching your pectorals, this exercise strengthens your rhomboids in the middle of your back. It also increases extension throughout your mid-back.

If you are doing this stretch while seated and your chair back is low enough, arch your back over the chair back as you squeeze your shoulder blades together. Hold for five, deep slow breaths.

You may feel or hear a few pops in your mid-back with this stretch, which is a good thing! It means your body is self-adjusting. If the relief from this self-adjustment lasts less than an hour, you still have a restricted joint in that area that didn't pop. If you feel this tension and lack of relief, I would advise seeing a chiropractor to get the restricted joints professionally released.

A Standing Version of the Pectoral Stretch

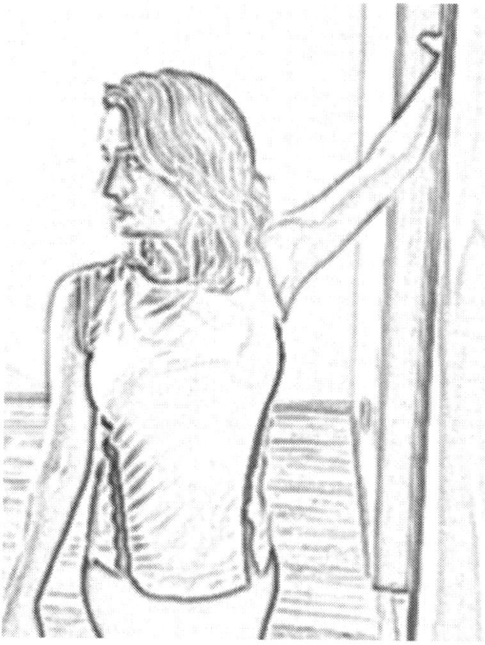

Figure 10-10

In this variation of the pectoral stretch, you stretch the pectoral muscles by standing in a doorway, placing your left palm against the doorframe with your arm at a 45-degree angle upward, and leaning into the doorway to open up the left chest (Figure 10-10). To add a stretch to your anterior neck muscles, turn your head to the right (away from the raised arm). Repeat on the other side.

This is a great stretch to relieve shoulder pain, pain down the arm, swelling of the arm and hands, and upper back pain.

Standing-in-Doorway Shoulder Stretches

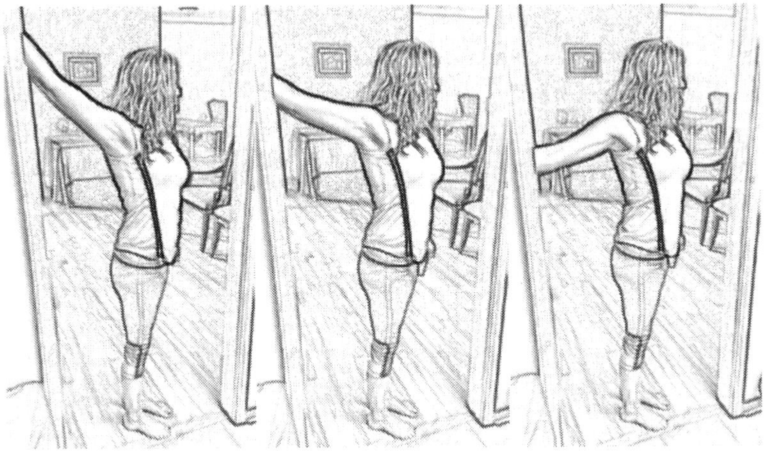

Figure 10-11: Pectoral stretch with arms at various heights to stretch different muscle fibers in the anterior shoulder and chest.

You can loosen up the muscles surrounding the shoulders further by doing the doorway stretch with your arm at a steeper angle above and below your shoulder (Figure 10-11). Varying the angle of the stretch allows you to stretch the various muscles of the anterior shoulder. It is a good way to warm up for the next stretch of the lateral chest muscles.

Wall Arm Stretch

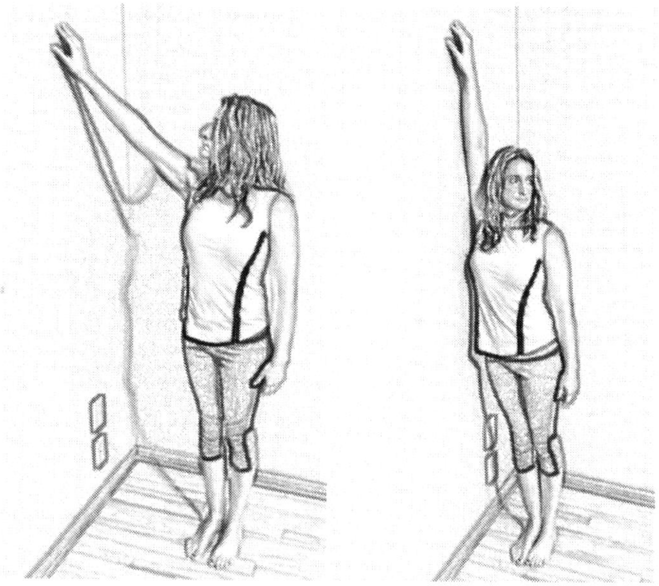

Figure 10-12: Shoulder stretch walking hands up the wall and then leaning into the wall to deepen the stretch.

Shoulders tend to tighten and lose their flexibility in abduction, limiting the range of motion of raising your arm above the horizon. A stiff shoulder leads to a stiff neck. Combat this by periodically raising your arms high above your head.

If you have difficulty raising your arms, walk your hand up a wall (Figure 10-12). Then lean into your arm against the wall to assist the stretch. Be careful not to hurt your shoulder. If you feel a stretch, you are improving your range of motion. If you feel a strain, you are harming your shoulder.

Arm-Across-Body Stretch

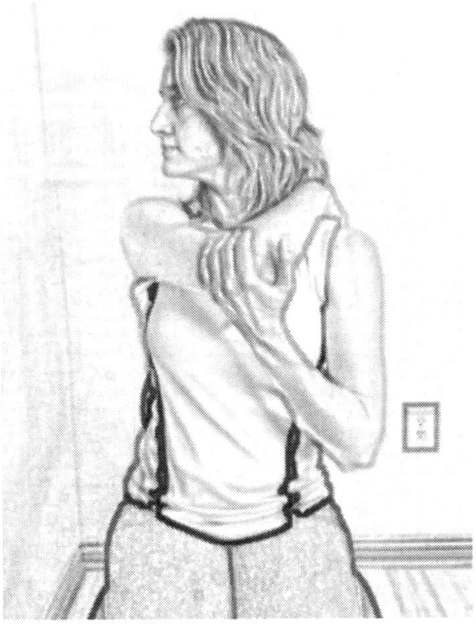

Figure 10-13

This stretch works the posterior shoulder muscles. Begin by pulling your right arm across your body with your left hand just above the right elbow (Figure 10-13). Rest your right hand behind your left shoulder. The farther you bring the right elbow toward your left shoulder, the deeper the stretch in your shoulder. You may even feel the upper back muscles stretching, which is good as long as you don't stretch to the point of pain and strain.

The shoulder is a very complicated joint with multiple small muscles that work together to move the shoulder in many different directions. Feel free to explore different angles of stretches by raising and lowering the elbow as you bring it across; this stretches different groups of muscles in the back of the shoulder and back.

You can add to this stretch by pressing your right elbow into your left hand, causing an isometric contraction of the muscles in the back of your upper right arm. Hold this contraction for three slow breaths, then relax your right arm and use your left hand to bring your right arm deeper into the stretch cautiously (do not pull too hard because you can overstretch the muscles). Repeat this up to three times. After releasing, rotate your shoulders a few times to help fully release the stretch. Then repeat on the other side.

Triceps and Lateral Body Stretch

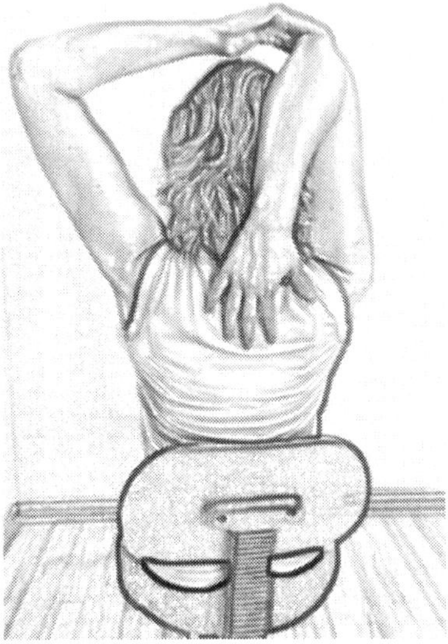

Figure 10-14

This stretch works the muscles in the back of your arm and those down the side of your torso. To perform the stretch, lift your right arm up, then bend your elbow so your right hand is dangling behind your head (Figure 10-14). Use your left hand to gently pull your right elbow even farther behind your head. Hold for three breaths. Do not overstretch. If you feel a painful strain, then you are literally straining your muscles and/or spraining your shoulder, potentially causing damage. Repeat on the other side.

This stretch is best done while standing, but it can be done in a seated position.

Cow Face Pose (a Deeper Triceps Stretch)

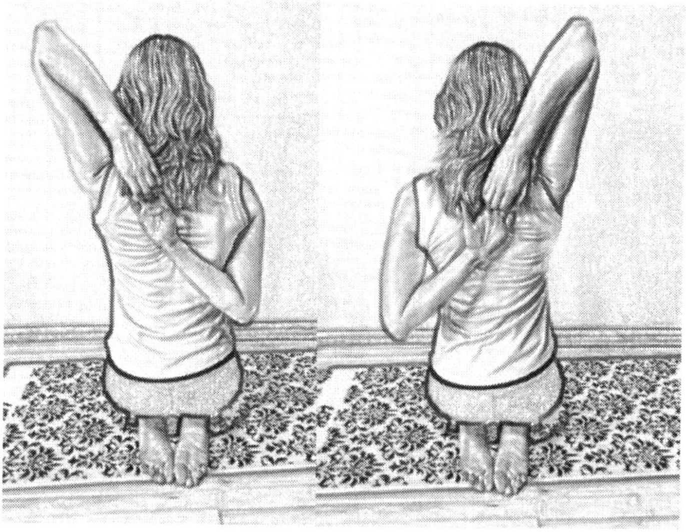

Figure 10-15

The cow face pose (also known as Apley's stretch) is another stretch that is easily done throughout the day. The stretch requires you to reach for your hands behind your back, which helps improve both your posture and the flexibility of the mid-back.

Reach your left hand up and over your left shoulder while reaching your right hand behind your back from below. Try to grab your right hand with your left hand (Figure 10-15). Hold your position for a few breaths and then switch your arm positions.

If you can't reach your fingers, modify the stretch using a towel or strap (Figure 10-16). If you use a strap, be careful that you don't overstretch. Listen to the limitations of your body.

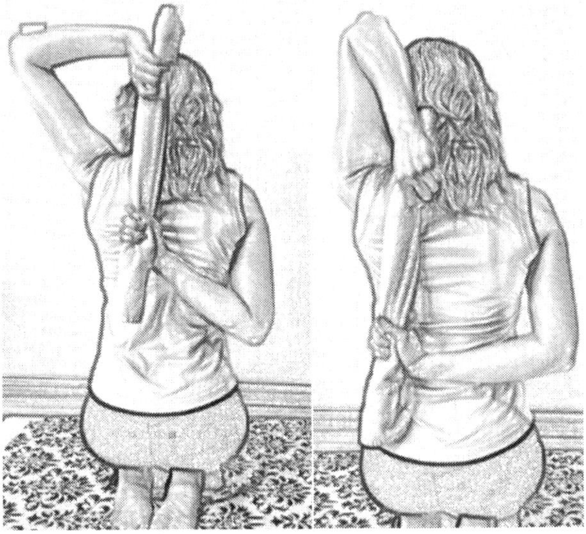

Figure 10-16: Modified cow face pose with strap.

You can watch my YouTube video for a more detailed explanation of how to go from a modified cow face pose to the full pose using the post-isometric technique on my YouTube Channel: www.youtube.com/channel/UC0dGeIPJ00LOLFIiXHAst8Q

Chapter 11: EXERCISES THAT HELP WITH NECK PAIN

AGAIN, MOST NECK PAIN involves tight neck muscles in the back of the neck (the posterior muscles), weak muscles between the shoulder blades (the rhomboids), and tight pectoral muscles (the muscles in the chest). This chapter shows you how to strengthen those weak rhomboids and posterior neck muscles

Isometric Exercises for the Neck

Many of these exercises use isometric contraction; that is, you contract your muscles without allowing movement. Think about pushing a car. Your arm muscles contract as you push the car, but your muscles aren't actually moving. The strain you feel in your muscles are isometric contractions. You want to try to achieve the same feeling when you do isometric exercises for your neck.

These neck exercises can be done while you are seated or standing. I suggest you stand if you can to increase blood flow and oxygenate your system.

Isometric Contraction in Flexion

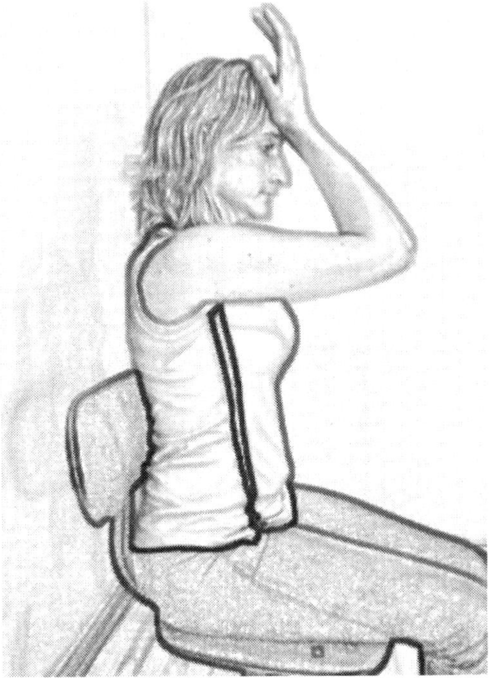

Figure 11-1

To do an isometric contraction for the muscles in the front of your neck (the anterior muscles), put your hands on your forehead (Figure 11-1). Press into your hands with your anterior neck muscles, but stop your head from moving with your hands. Hold for three breaths. This strengthens the anterior neck muscles.

Isometric Contraction in Rotation

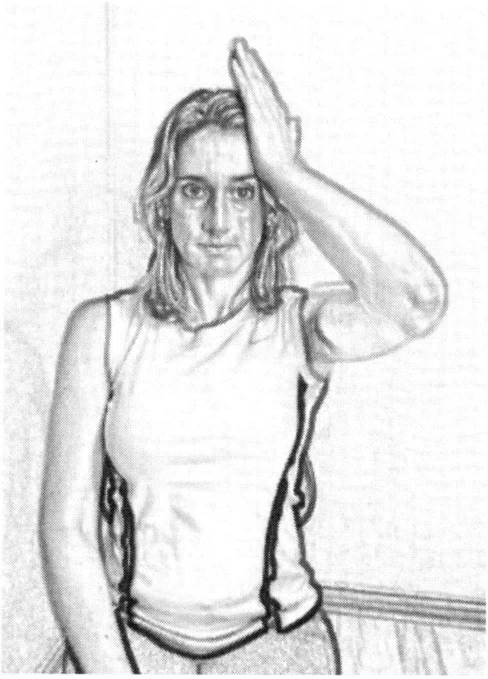

Figure 11-2

To do an isometric contraction for the muscles at the sides of your neck, put your right hand at the right side of your forehead (Figure 11-2). Press into it by trying to turn your head to the right, but use your hand to prevent the rotation. This exercises the rotation muscles in your neck. Hold for three breaths. Repeat on the left side.

Isometric Contraction in Lateral Flexion

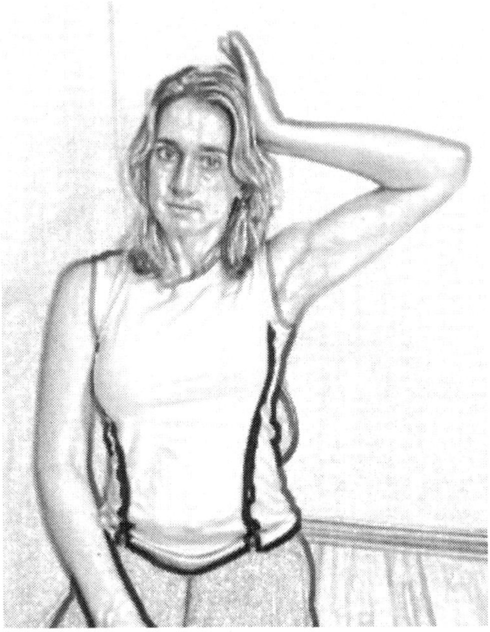

Figure 11-3

Put your hand to the right side of your head (Figure 11-3). Press into it by laterally flexing your head to the right, but prevent your head from moving by applying pressure with your hand. This exercises the lateral flexion muscles in your neck. Hold for three breaths. Repeat on the left side.

Post-Isometric Contractions for the Neck

Post-isometric stretching involves bringing a muscle to a stretched position, then contracting the muscle at 30 to 50 percent of its strength without allowing it to move for three to five slow breaths. On the last exhale, you relax the muscle, allowing it to lengthen farther, deepening the stretch. When you contract opposing muscle groups, you fool them into thinking they are in a contracted (shortened) state, so when they relax, they elongate, allowing for a deeper stretch. You can repeat this up to three times.

Unlike the isometric contractions on the previous pages, in the following exercises you stretch one set of neck muscles and then contract the opposing muscle group without allowing the muscles to move by placing a hand against your head.

Post-isometric stretches can be performed with any muscle to increase flexibility. Football players often stretch their hamstrings using isometric contractions.

Post-Isometric Contraction in Rotation

To stretch the neck in rotation with a post-isometric contraction, turn your head as far to the left as is comfortable (Figure 11-4).

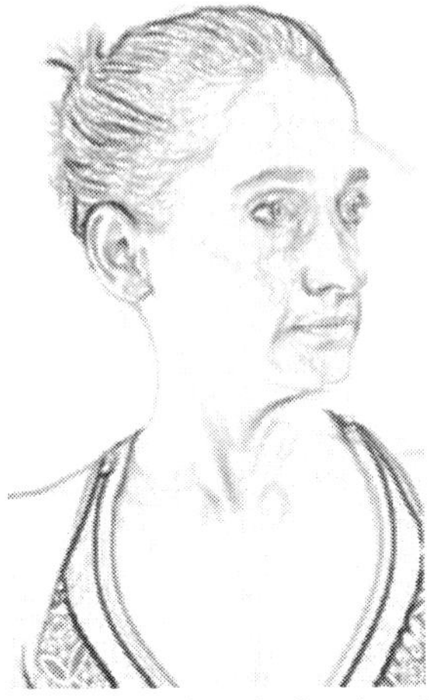

Figure 11-4: Turning the head to the left.

You (or your practitioner) place a hand on your right temporal region to provide resistance as you press into the hand as if you are trying to turn your head to the right (Figure 11-5).

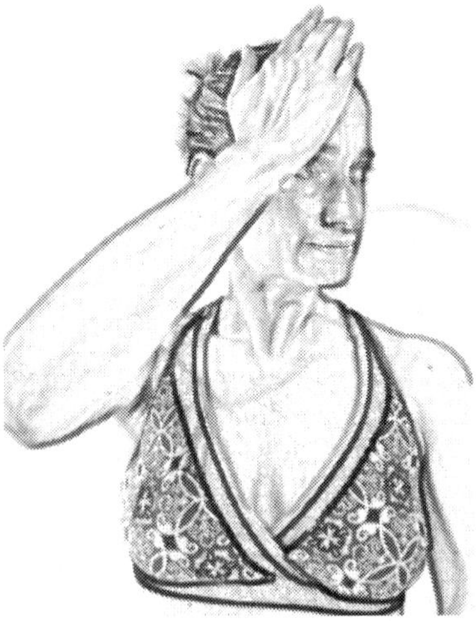

Figure 11-5: Isometric contraction to the right (providing resistance with the right hand).

Hold this contracted isometric state for three to five deep, slow breaths. You (or your practitioner) should not push your head to the left because this can strain the muscles. On the last exhale, relax, allowing your head to turn farther to the left (Figure 11-6).

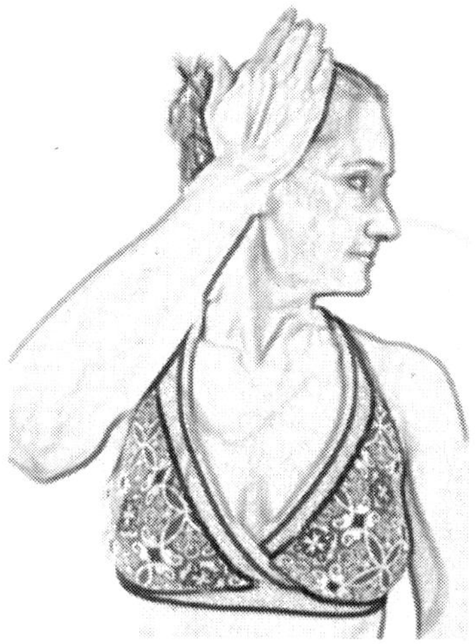

Figure 11-6: Turning the head farther to the left without pressing with the right hand.

When you've reached your comfortable limit in left rotation, you (or your practitioner) provide resistance as you turn your head to the right again and as you (or they) resist by pressing to the left (Figure 11-7).

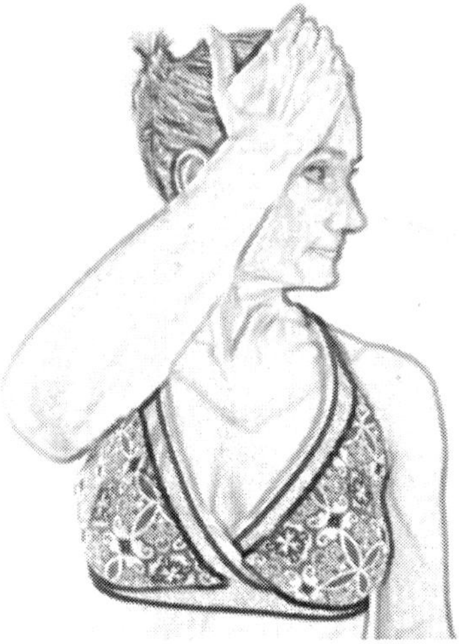

Figure 11-7: Pressing into the hand to the right a second time.

Again, this is an isometric contraction, so your head shouldn't turn at all. Just try to turn your head to the right as you (or your practitioner) hold your head still. Hold for three to five breaths and then relax. If you can turn farther to the left, do so, repeating the isometric contraction to the right again.

Repeat up to three times in one direction. Then repeat, turning your head to the right, with isometrics to the left.

Post-Isometric Contraction in Lateral Flexion

Post-isometric stretching can be used for lateral flexion as well. First, tilt you head as far as you can to the right (Figure 11-8).

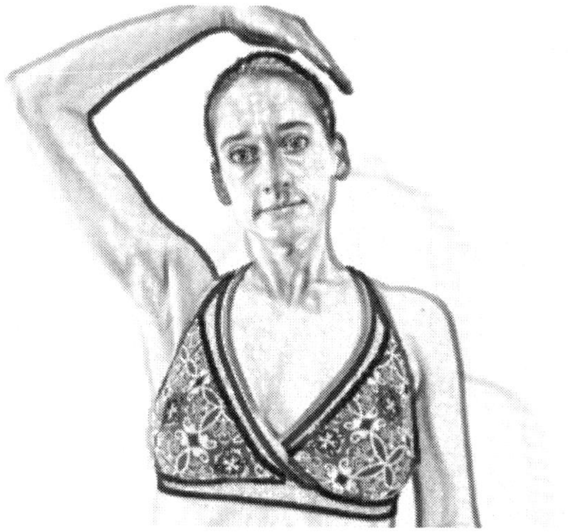

Figure 11-8: Tilting the head to the right.

Then place your right hand on the left side of the top of your head and press your head into your hand (Figure 11-9), contracting the muscles that would tilt your head to the left).

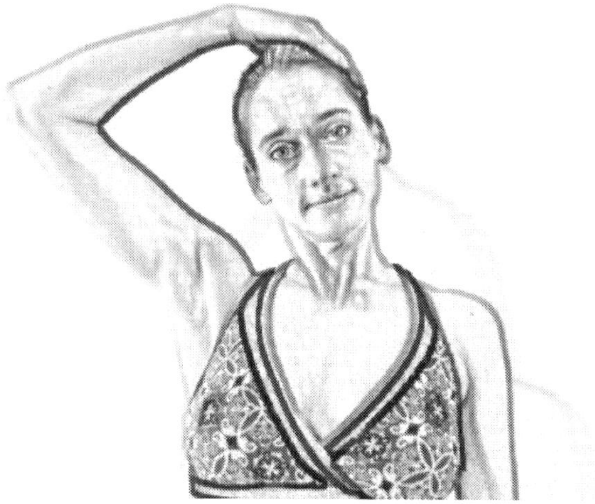

Figure 11-9: Isometric contraction of the neck to the left.

Hold the contraction for three breaths. On the third exhale, relax and see if your head will fall into a deeper tilt to the right (Figure 11-10).

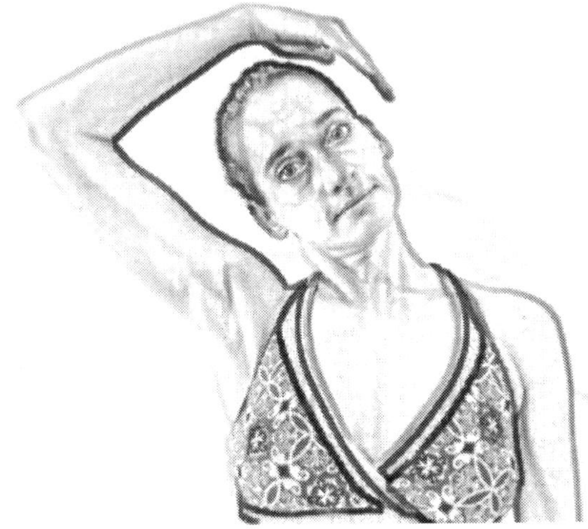

Figure 11-10: Going deeper into the stretch.

If you can't go deeper, just press into the right hand again. If your head tilted farther to the right, bring your right hand to the left side of the head again and press into it (Figure 11-11).

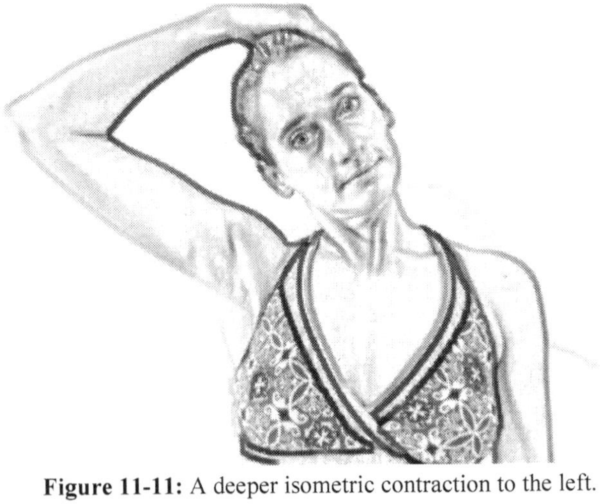

Figure 11-11: A deeper isometric contraction to the left.

Again, hold for three breaths and relax on the final exhale. Repeat this up to three times.

Then repeat on the other side.

You can do post-isometric stretches throughout the day. To learn how, visit my YouTube channel and watch: https://www.youtube.com/watch?v=PDcFpJuEoTg

Strong Posterior Neck Stretch

This particular stretch isn't necessarily good for everyone. Please confirm with your healthcare provider that this stretch is appropriate for you.

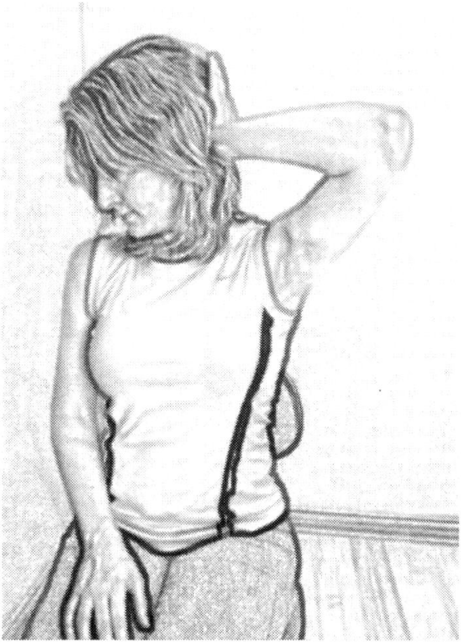

Figure 11-12

To work the muscles in the front and the back of your neck at the same time, try this exercise. Turn your head about halfway toward your right shoulder. Place your left hand at the base of your skull with the base of your thumb where your skull rests on your spine. Tuck your chin in and press back with your head as you press forward and upward with your left hand (Figure 11-12).

This combination forms a strong traction for the muscles in

the back of your neck on the left and strengthens the muscles in the front of your neck on the right.

Repeat on the other side.

Rhomboid Strengthening Exercise

Rhomboids are the muscles between your shoulder blades. You can strengthen them by simply squeezing your shoulder blades back and down as if you're bringing the bottom of your shoulder blades together (Figure 11-13). Hold this position for a couple of breaths. Remember to keep your shoulders back and *down* as you do this exercise. It is more important to do this exercise frequently throughout the day instead of focusing on the number of times you do it in a row. Try doing this stretch every twenty minutes.

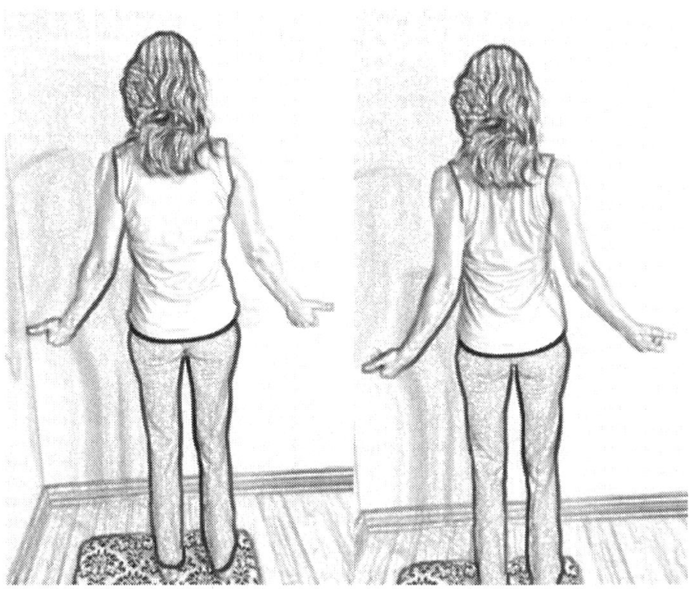

Figure 11-13: Strengthen the rhomboids by squeezing the shoulder blades back and down.

If your pectoral muscles (the muscles in your chest) are tight and/or overdeveloped, they will pull your shoulders forward and cause you to slouch, which can lead to neck pain. Doing this rhomboid strengthening exercise will not only strengthen these opposing back muscles, but it will also stretch out your tight pectoral muscles and make it easier for you to stand up straight.

Be careful not to engage your upper back muscles (the trapezius muscles). They tend to be overdeveloped and want to assist your weaker rhomboid muscles (Figure 11-14).

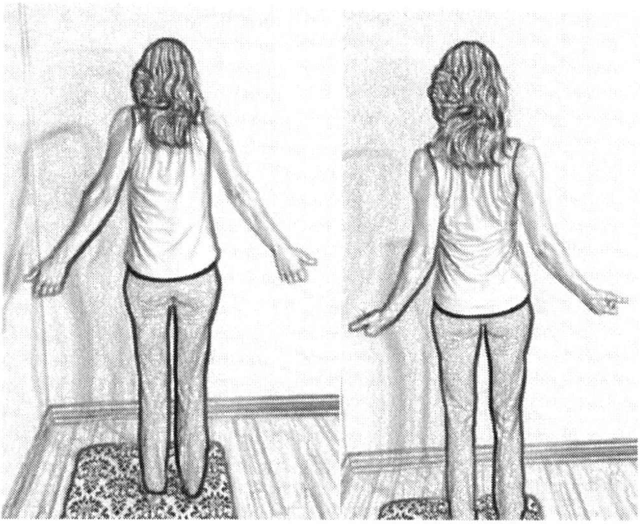

Figure 11-14: Incorrect shoulder squeeze (left) versus proper shoulder squeeze.

Rhomboid Pull

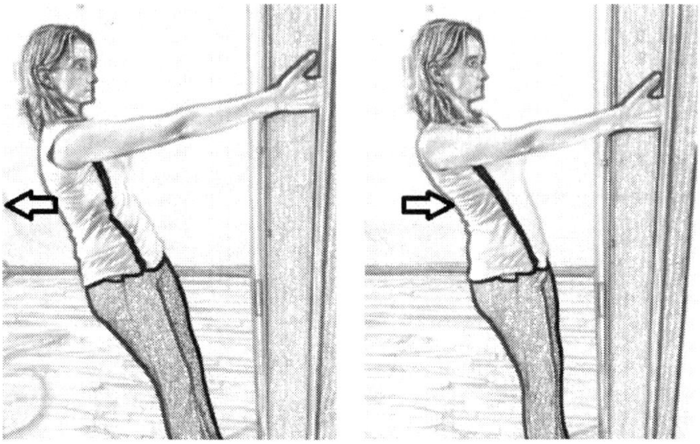

Figure 11-15

Grab onto a doorframe with one hand and lean back (keep your shoulders down, away from your ears). Then pull your weight up by squeezing your shoulders back and down by contracting your rhomboids (Figure 11-15). Be careful not to pull yourself up with your arm muscles — that's cheating! Then relax, allowing your body to lean back. Repeat ten times.

Repeat on the opposite side.

Shoulder Squeeze

If you want to make the shoulder squeeze a heavy-duty workout, add an exercise band (Figure 11-16).

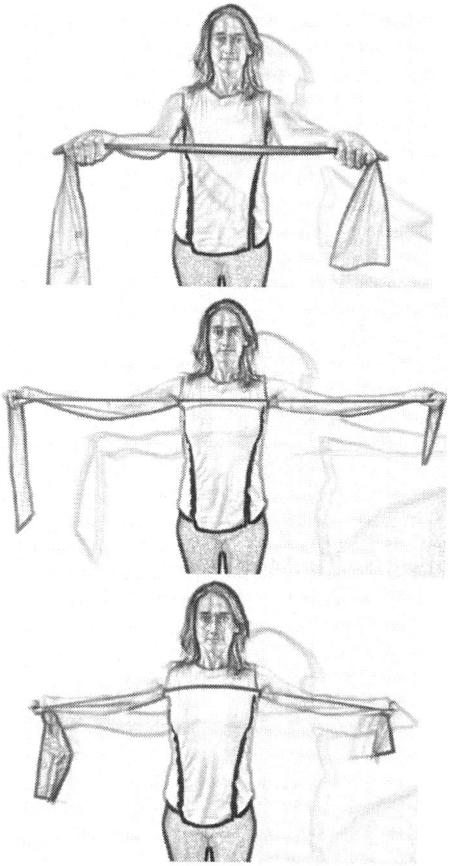

Figure 11-16: Rhomboid strengthening with an exercise band.

I recommend doing this exercise with your palms up because it helps the shoulder blades maintain a better position. It also changes the orientation of your palms, which are usually facedown with regular daily activities. Remember, if you do too much of one thing, you should balance it out with the opposite action every once in a while.

Chapter 12: TIGHTENING YOUR ABS

THIS chapter shows how I have modified crunches to really target the abdominal muscles while protecting the neck.

I have already gone over how to strengthen the back muscles and the anterior neck muscles and how to stretch the chest and shoulder muscles. Now I want to show you how to strengthen your core muscles so you can have better posture throughout the day, which will help keep your neck healthy over time.

My Favorite Routine to Tighten the Abs

I believe the best way to strengthen the core muscles is by slowly contracting the abdominal muscles (otherwise known as doing crunches) with very little movement as you exhale. If you are doing core-strengthening crunches correctly, it won't look like you are doing much because core muscles are stabilizers more than movers. But when you do these exercises correctly, you may shake with the effort. If you are moving a lot, you are likely doing the moves incorrectly by engaging the muscles involved with movement (like the hip flexors).

I outline the steps of my favorite core workout here, but you can also watch a demonstration of the workout online at https://youtu.be/5EAqQ4B7X0Y.

- First, lay on your back.

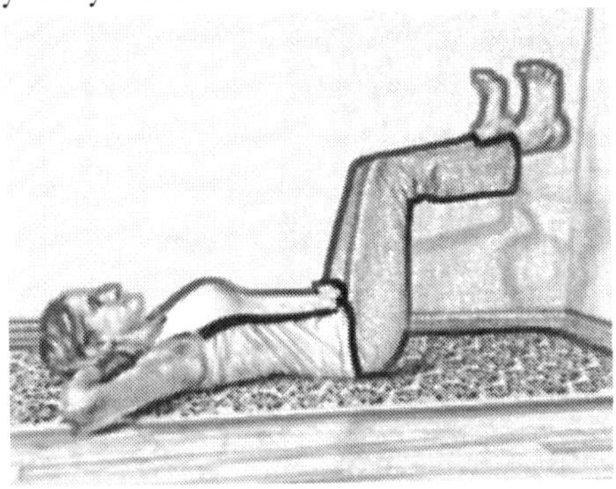

Figure 12-1: Starting position for a crunch.

- Bring your hips, knees, and ankles to 90 degrees (Figure 12-1). To make it easier, you can rest your legs on a chair or keep your feet on the floor.
- Keep your knees and ankles apart. To make it harder, bring your knees closer together—but not touching—and make sure your ankles are spread farther apart than your knees.
- Put your hands behind your head. To make it easier, put your hands palm-down on the floor with your arms along your sides or your hands on your stomach so you can feel the muscles contracting (Figure 12-2).

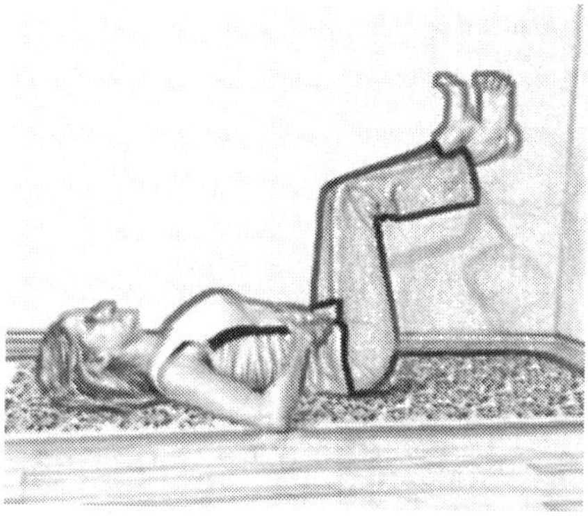

Figure 12-2: Alternate starting position for a crunch: Keep your head down so you don't have to support the neck, and place your hands on your stomach to see if you are contracting the correct muscles.

- Look up at the ceiling but keep your chin tucked toward your chest. This keeps space between the bones of your neck and helps prevent you from straining your neck.
- Inhale.
- As you exhale, contract your stomach (rectus abdominis muscle), which should press your back to the floor and lift your pubic bone toward your chest (Figure 12-3). This is where most people make the mistake of moving too much. If your knees move a lot closer to your head, you are likely engaging the wrong muscles (your hip flexors instead of your abdominal muscles). Abdominal muscles are stabilizers, not movers.

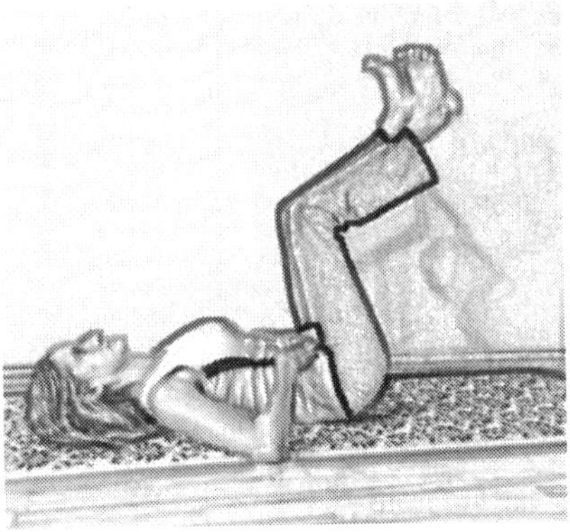

•

Figure 12-3: Exhale and contract your lower abdominal muscles, causing your pubic bone to move toward your sternum and your pelvic bone to tilt, raising your buttocks slightly off the floor.

- If you have neck pain, *do not* lift your head during abdominal contractions as in Figure 12-4.

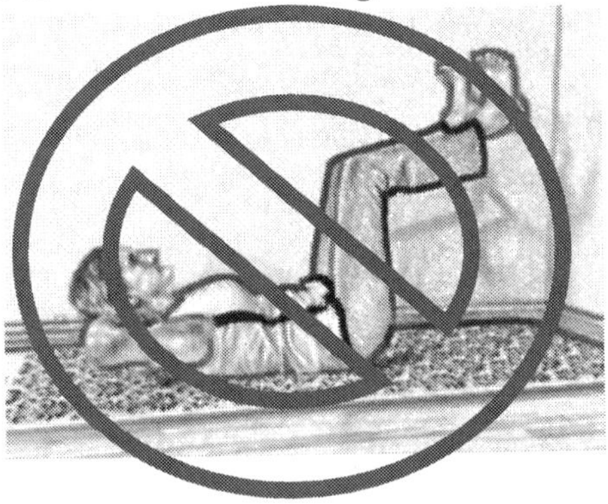

Figure 12-4: Do not lift your head while doing crunches if you have neck pain.

- As you inhale, relax your stomach so you can expand your diaphragm (Figure 12-5). Don't relax so much that your back arches off the ground. Your stomach should expand outward so your diaphragm has room to expand down, but your back should not arch.

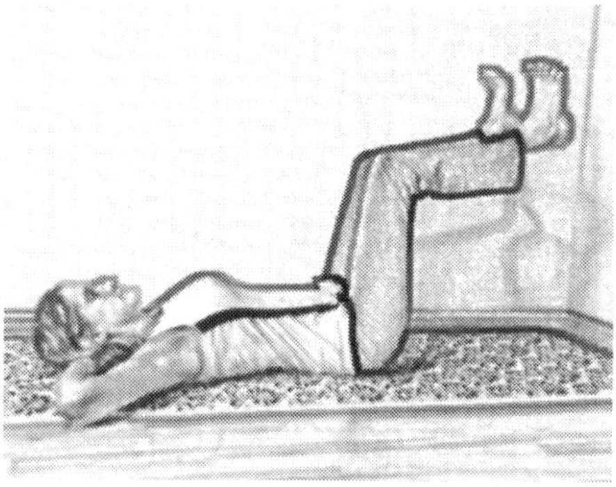

Figure 12-5: Expand your belly as you inhale.

- Repeat the exhale/contract, inhale/relax cycle up to ten times, depending on your core strength.

Note: If you work your abdominal muscles too hard, they may not be able to contract completely the next day, making you vulnerable to blowing out your back. I have had too many patients report that a day or two after an intense workout (be it in the gym or their garden), they bent over to pick up a light object (like a pen) and blew out their back. This is because they weren't expecting to have to purposely engage their core to protect their back for such a mundane movement. Because their core muscles were fatigued, the weight of their body leaning over with their arms extended was enough to sprain the discs in their lower back. If you try this core workout routine, limit yourself to a couple of repetitions at first and see how you feel in the next day or two. If everything is okay, you can add more repetitions. Go slowly and give yourself the time it takes to strengthen your muscles.

Working Out the Obliques

After you've done some crunches, you can work to strengthen the muscles that run along the sides of your torso.

- To work out your right abdominal oblique muscles (the muscles in the side wall of your belly between your lower ribs and pelvic bone on the right), lie on your back with your knees bent at 90 degrees with knees and ankles apart. Breathe in and twist your pelvis slightly to the left (Figure 12-6).

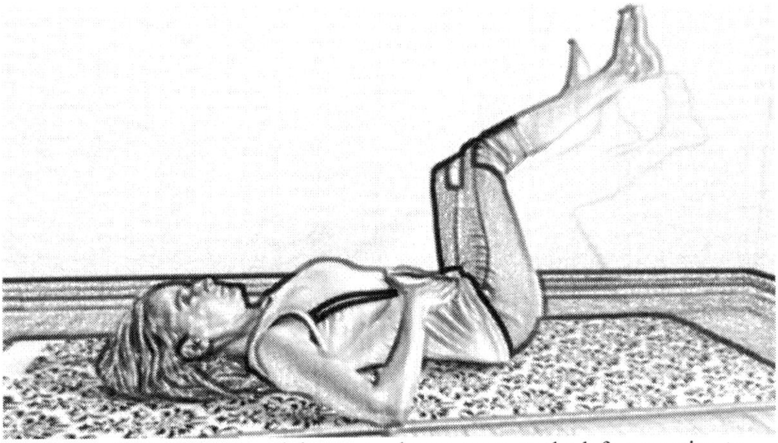

Figure 12-6: Tilt your pelvis so your knees move to the left, preparing to exercise the right abdominal oblique muscles.

When you contract your right abdominal muscles, *do not lift your head* (you may strain your neck; Figure 12-7).

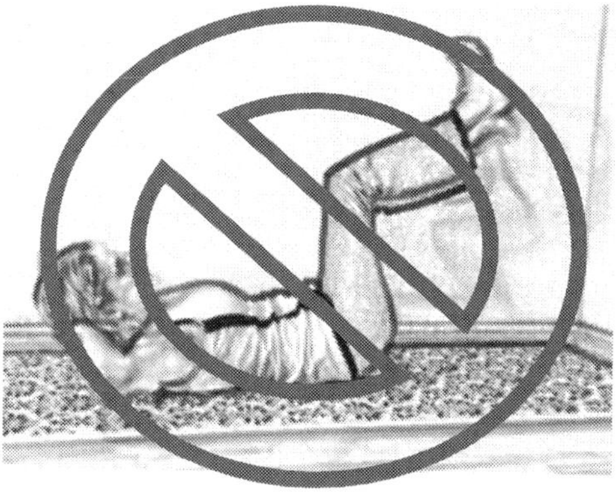

Figure 12-7: If you have neck pain, do not lift your head because it can further strain your neck!

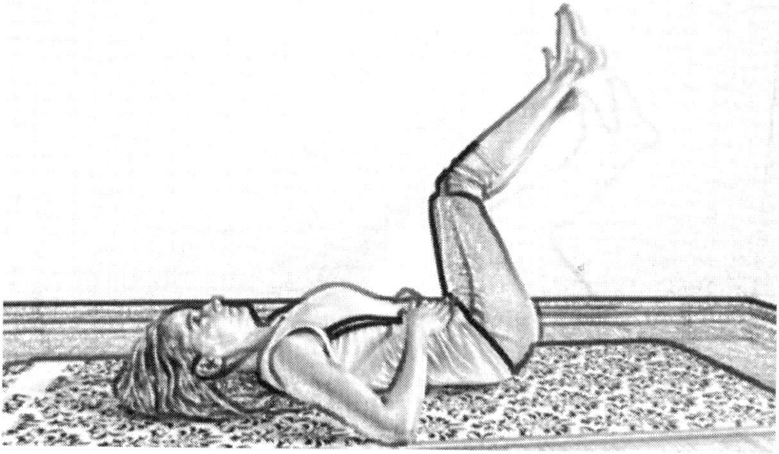

Figure 12-8: Contract the right oblique muscles and bring the right pelvic bone toward the left chest.

- Exhale and contract your right abdominal oblique muscles. This should lift the right pelvic bone (the ilium) toward the left lower ribs. The left lower ribs, chest, and shoulder may even rise off the floor. The goal is not to bring the left shoulder to the right knee; the goal is to contract the correct muscle. The right oblique abdominal muscle is not connected to the left shoulder or right leg, so if either is moving, you are engaging the wrong muscles. Keep the left shoulder away from the right knee and the left shoulder out of your peripheral vision.

- Repeat the exhale/contract, inhale/relax cycle up to ten times, depending on your core strength.
- Then switch sides. While inhaling, twist your pelvis (still bent at 90 degrees with knees and ankles apart) slightly to the right (lowering your legs slightly to the right this time).
- Exhale and contract your left abdominal oblique muscles. This should lift the left pelvic bone (the ilium) toward the right lower ribs.
- Repeat the exhale/contract, inhale/relax cycle up to ten times, depending on your core strength.

Stretching the Abdominal Muscles

It's a good idea to stretch your abdominal muscles after you've finished your strengthening exercises. Here's how.

- Lie on your back and put your feet on the floor, hip width apart.
- Bring your arms to your sides, palms down, and tuck your shoulders slightly in and underneath you so you can lift your pelvis up into a bridge pose (Figure 12-9).

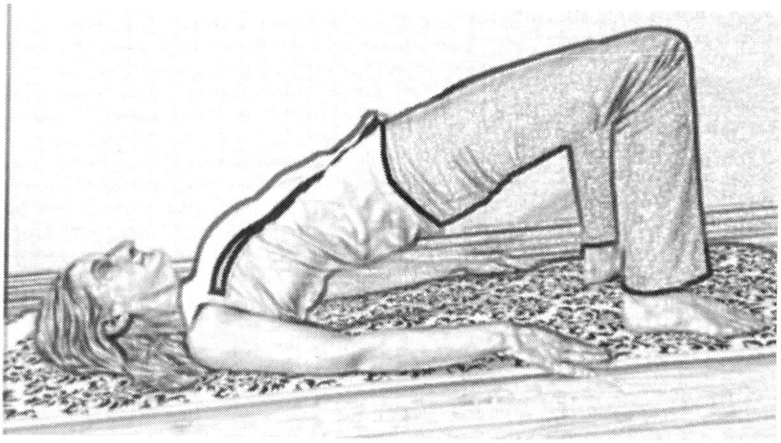

• **Figure 12-9:** Bridge pose (an active back bend).

- Hold for up to ten slow inhale-exhale cycles. Feel free to do full wheel pose instead if able (see Chapter 9).

Chapter 13: HOW TO TREAT FOR TRIGGER AND PRESSURE POINTS IN THE NECK AND UPPER BACK

PRESSURE POINTS are points on the body that you press to relieve a symptom. Trigger points are tender muscle spasms that can put pressure on a nerve, leading to pain in another area of the body.

In this chapter, I show trigger points and pressure points you can work on to see if it relieves your neck pain. But it is best to get a professional massage for your tight muscles. A good massage therapist, chiropractor, physical therapist, or other healthcare provider who specializes in releasing muscle spasms can find all of your tight muscles and trigger points and work them out.

Receiving a professional massage is better than self-massage because it is easier to get your muscles to relax when you're not activating them while massaging them.

The professional performing your massage should have professional myofascial releasing tools like the T-bar, Graston instruments, and other powerful massage tools like the Thumper Maxi Pro Massager, the Jeanie Rub massager, and

Rapid Release Technology (RRT; see Chapter 18 for more about this device) to name a few.

Personally, I aim to get at least one massage a month, and then I maintain the benefits of the massage with daily self-massage between my professional massage appointments.

Trigger Points in Your Neck and Shoulders

You may find tender, bumpy spots at the base of your skull (suboccipitals; Figure 13-1), along the ropey muscles in the front of your neck (SCM, anterior scalenes; Figure 13-1), or along the posterior neck muscles or the upper back (trapezius muscles and levator scapulae muscles; Figure 13-2). When you find one of these spots, lightly press on it to see if it increases your neck pain. If pressing on the spot increases your neck pain, it is likely the cause of your neck pain.

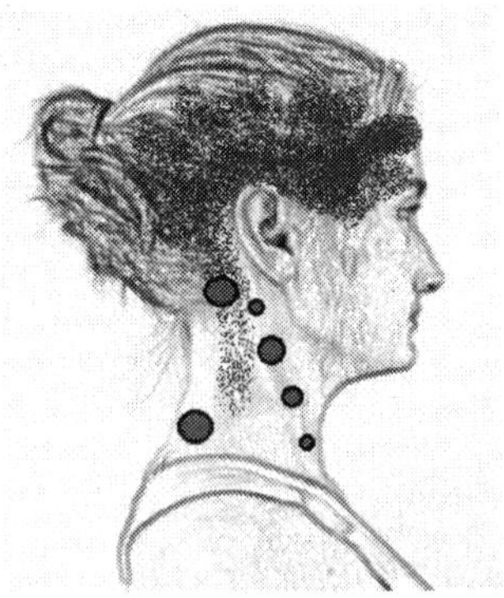

Figure 13-1: Trigger points in the SCM and trapezius muscles.

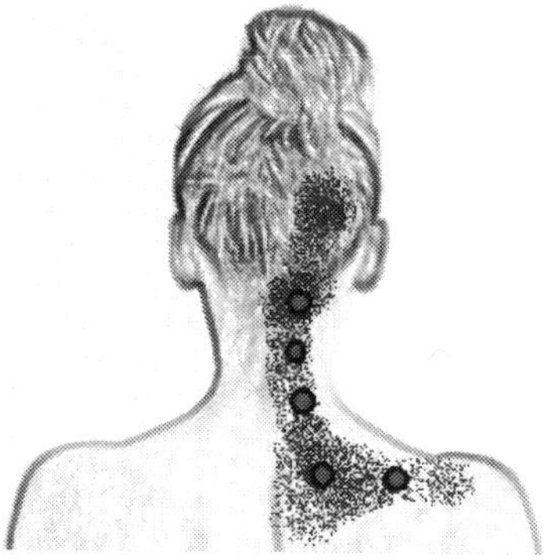

Figure 13-2: More trigger points in the trapezius and levator scapulae muscles.

To treat these points, hold the pressure for three breaths (Figures 13-3 and 13-4). This helps squeeze out the metabolic waste trapped in the chronically contracted muscle. When you let go, new blood will flow into the muscle, bringing in nutrients and allowing the muscle to relax. When the muscle relaxes, it takes pressure off the nerves or blood vessels that are referring pain into your neck.

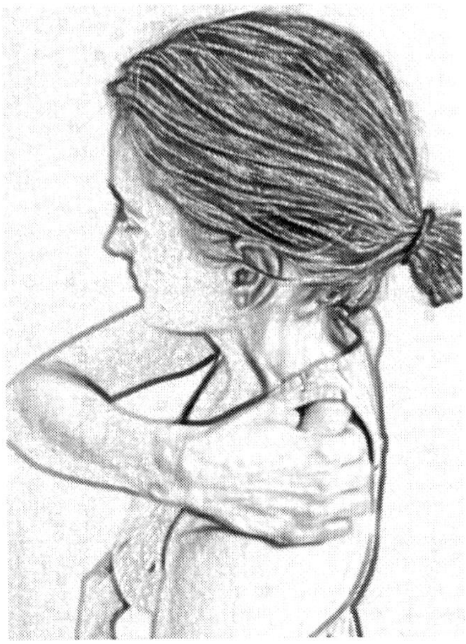

Figure 13-3: Self-massaging the upper part of the trapezius muscle.

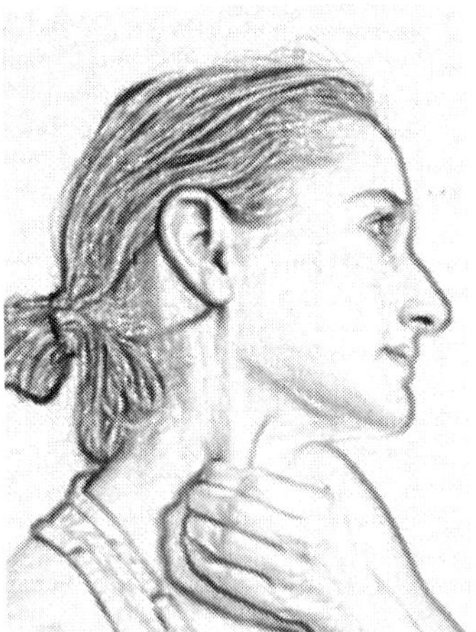

Figure 13-4: Self-massaging the SCM (an anterior neck muscle).

If the muscle is still tight and sore, you can repeat this up to three times several times a day.

You may experience immediate relief from your neck pain after working on your pressure points. Sometimes it may take a couple of days before you notice relief.

When massaging your extremities, like your forearms and hands, always press harder on the stroke up (toward the heart) and lighter on the stroke down (away from the heart; Figure 13-5). That way, you assist the lymphatic and vascular drainage. If you stroke firmly away from your heart, you may hinder this drainage and cause swelling of the fingers and hands.

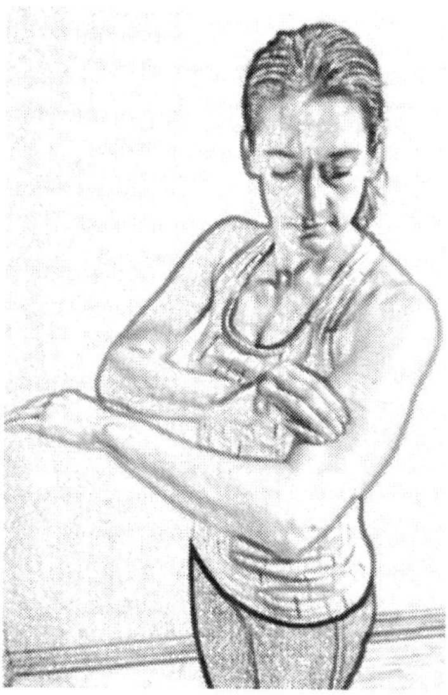

Figure 13-5: Self-massaging by stroking up the arm toward the heart to help lymph drain.

To learn more about the lymphatic system, check out my books *Combat Slouching* and *Top Seven Ways to Combat the Effects of Sitting*.

If your neck pain is not responding to your treatment, or if it is worsening in any way, see your healthcare provider.

Self-Massage Tools

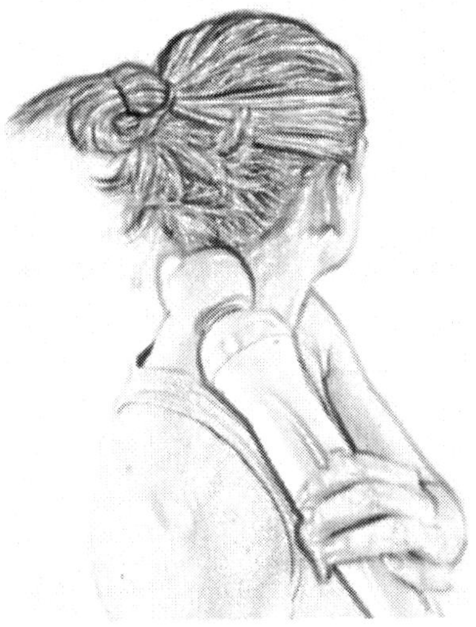

Figure 13-6: Performing self-massage with a long-handled, vibrating device.

To increase the benefits of a professional massage, it helps to self-massage at home between your professional massages. Otherwise, after only a few days, your muscles may tense back up from your routine activities. If you massage your muscles daily, the benefits of the professional massage will last that much longer.

Many devices at a wide range of price points are available to help you self-massage. I prefer vibrating massage tools with a long handle to make reaching the back of the neck and upper back easier (Figure 13-6). Such tools run from as little as $30 to hundreds of dollars.

I also recommend tools like the Thera Cane and Body Back Buddy (Figure 13-7). They help you press on trigger points in the back of your torso and neck while keeping your arms down, which allows the upper back muscles to stay relaxed. The cost of each tool is about $40.

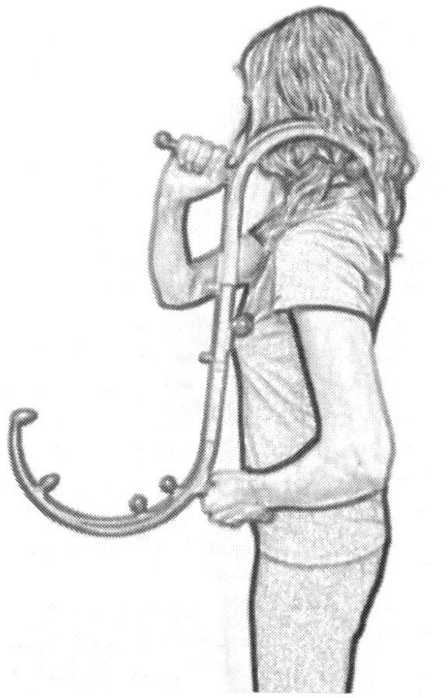

Figure 13-7: Body Back Buddy.

But no self-massage is better than a professional massage. If you suffer from neck pain, consider treating yourself to regular professional massages. I like to go at least once a month because I have a physical job. If you sit at a computer all day, it is important to stretch regularly and treat yourself to massage at least once a month as well.

If you find the relief you get from a professional massage does not last more than a day or two, try chiropractic and/or acupuncture. If a chiropractor just stretches your joints, yet doesn't release your muscle tension, your bones will become restricted with the constant pressures exerted on them. This is why I prefer practitioners that marry these techniques with massage or Gua Sha.

Chapter 14: TO TAKE OR NOT TO TAKE PAIN PILLS?

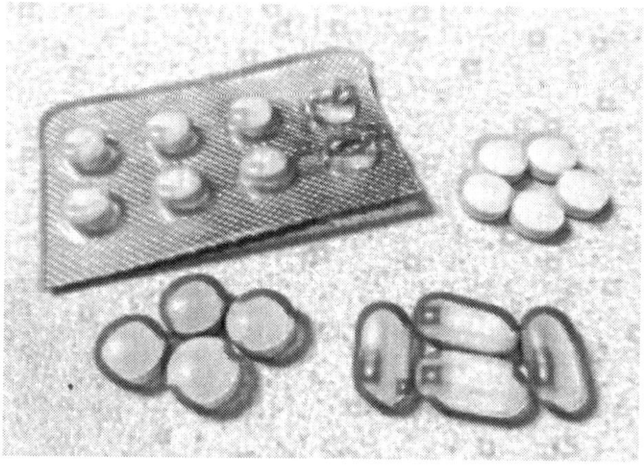

IF YOU TAKE PAIN PILLS for every neck pain, this chapter is for you. Almost every one of my books contains this chapter. I can't stress enough how taking pain relievers on a regular basis is not healthy in the long run. Still, I often hear from new patients that they take over-the-counter pain relievers almost every day for their neck pain!

After they learn to move their body more often throughout the day, eat healthier, avoid their personal triggers, and get more sleep, they often find they no longer need to take pain relievers. I hope the advice in this book helps you feel well enough that you no longer need pain medication!

Why an Easy Solution Can Be Harmful

When people have neck pain, the first thing they usually reach for is an everyday painkiller like aspirin. However, nonsteroidal anti-inflammatory drugs (NSAIDs), like acetaminophen or aspirin, are not as safe to take as many people think. Such drugs have side effects and are very hard on the liver and kidneys, and can lead to organ failure and early death.

Indeed, I know people who take several OTC (over-the-counter) pain relievers every day and have for years. But some people get away with smoking for years, too, and never develop cancer or COPD (chronic obstructive pulmonary disease). This does not mean smoking is safe. In the same way, people who take pain relievers every day do so at a cost to their overall health.

Don't get me wrong. I'm grateful to have access to medicines; they definitely have their uses. But America has a problem with overprescribing drugs. As an example, 99 percent of the world's Vicodin is prescribed in the United States.[2]

I have treated many people who were taking so many medications that they had to keep a written list of them.

---

[2] Vicodin Addiction, "Nearly 100 Percent of the World's Vicodin Prescriptions Are Used in U.S."

Some of these drugs were prescribed to treat the side effects of the medications they were taking for their original complaint. Sadly, instead of curing their condition, the medications were muting the symptoms of their disease. After educating these patients about lifestyle changes and herbal remedies, I helped them get off many of their medications (with their medical doctor's approval).

Medication is great for the short term because it offers a quick fix, but long-term use of chemicals is unhealthy. Prolonged use of medication leads to a decrease in quality of life. Such patients may be living with less pain, but at what cost to their body?

Consider this startling statistic: "NSAID use causes nearly 103,000 hospitalizations and 16,500 deaths. More people die each year from NSAIDs-related complications than from AIDS and cervical cancer in the US."[3] Furthermore, I have had too many patients in their late sixties find out that they have stage three kidney failure because of their NSAID usage over the years. And I have known of too many people who have died of liver failure because of acetaminophen usage.[4]

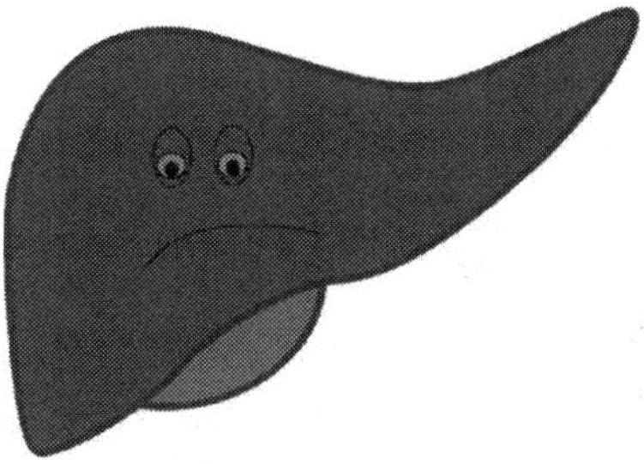

---

[3] American Gastroenterological Association, "Study Shows Long-term Use of NSAIDs Causes Severe Intestinal Damage."

[4] Zimmerman, "Drugs Used to Treat Rheumatic and Musculospastic Disease," *Hepatotoxicity*.

Why Avoiding Pain Relievers Is a Better Solution

So how do you balance the speed of pain relief that NSAIDs bring with their potential harmful effects? First, try other treatments to relieve your discomfort. If you take pain pills every day, their effectiveness wears off over time, and eventually you will have a difficult time overcoming the pain, even with pain relievers.

I do not believe in masking pain—we have pain for a reason. You do not want to turn off your body's alarm system. It would be like taking the battery out of the smoke detectors in your home so you don't have to listen to them beep as your house burns down.

When you start taking pain medication, your nerves are unnaturally suppressed. They then become more sensitive to irritations that cause pain once that suppression wears off. As a result, you lose your ability to naturally deal with pain, and you become more dependent on pain pills.

If you are not suffering from a traumatic injury but from chronic aches and pains, finding the root source of the pain and treating it through diet, stretches, and exercises instead of masking the pain is far healthier in the long run.

If you are taking pain relievers regularly, *stop*!

The fast and easy path for relieving neck pain is to take pain medication, but it is also the path to a shorter lifespan. If you take a pain pill for every ache, your body will adapt and be able to better process the pain medication, making it less effective for your pain. As a result, you will have to take stronger and stronger doses to achieve the same effect over time, harming your organs more and more until something fails and you become seriously ill and die before your time.

Yes, you will feel *awful* for a few weeks as you find other ways to treat your neck pain, but tough it out. Once your body re-acclimates to a healthier lifestyle, you will rarely be in pain, and even if you are in pain, you may not need pain relievers to alleviate it.

TOPICAL PAIN RELIEF FOR THE NECK AND ARMS

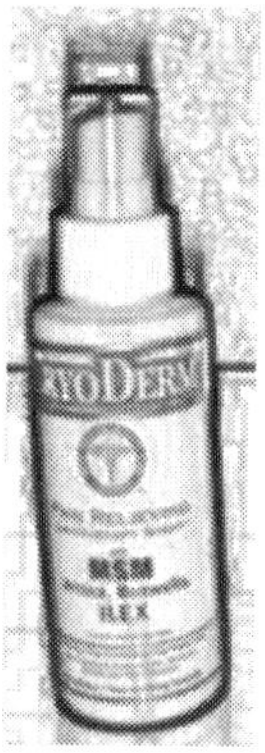

When your neck is in pain, instead of taking pain pills, think about applying a topical pain reliever. Why take a pill that affects your whole body and potentially harms your organs, when you can use a topical treatment that provides localized relief without the negative side effects of oral medication.

My favorite it Cryoderm. It is a cooling blend of menthol, arnica, and other herbs. It comes in spray, roll-on, and gel applications.

This may work to alleviate your pain enough, that it will help you wean off of your pain medication. If not, the following chapters have some other alternative you can try.

Chapter 15: ICE OR HEAT THERAPY FOR NECK PAIN

IF YOU ARE EXPERIENCING PAIN and are looking for an alternative to over-the-counter pain relievers, temperature therapy may be an option. Heat therapy and ice therapy are useful, and sometimes can be used interchangeably.

Heat Therapy

Heat is a great analgesic (pain reducer) and opens up capillary beds, bringing more blood to the region that is experiencing pain. This is great for tight muscles. However, heat therapy is also inflammatory. If your neck pain is caused by inflammation, heat can make it worse.

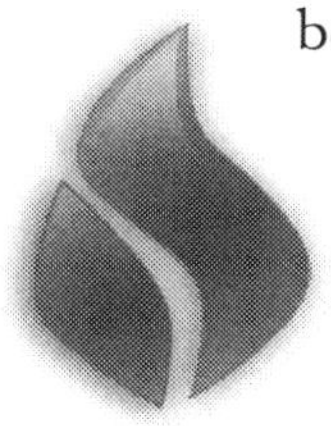

Ice Therapy

Like heat, ice is a great analgesic. But ice is also an anti-inflammatory. Ice therapy is a suitable treatment for acute injuries (during the inflamed state) because ice therapy causes your blood vessels to constrict, which reduces blood supply to the region. But if you don't have any inflammation, ice therapy is unhealthy for tissues already starved for blood, as with neck pain that is caused by spastic muscles.

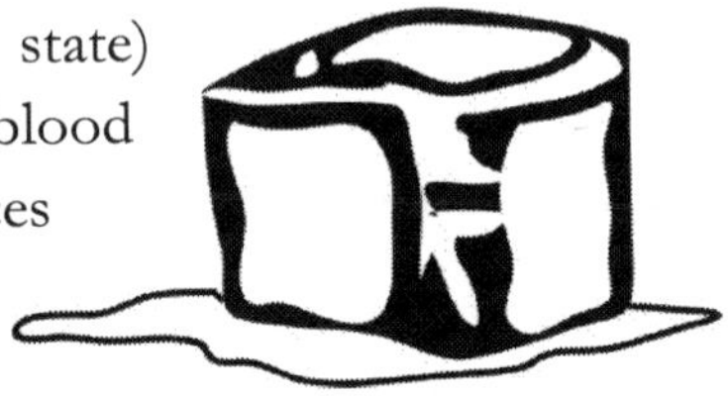

Careful!

Be careful with heat and ice. They are very effective tools when used correctly, but they can be dangerous when used incorrectly or to treat the wrong ailment.

Patients often make an emergency visit to my office after sleeping with a heating pad. This is a dangerous practice. It is too easy to overheat the region and wake up in a terribly inflamed state.

It is also dangerous to sleep with an ice pack, especially if you are on pain pills. I have had more than one patient wake up with frostbite under an ice pack after having slept with one.

The Safest Treatment for Neck Pain

I believe the safest self-treatment for most neck pain is to

1. Heat the upper back (trapezius region) for ten minutes to bring nutrient-filled blood to the area and to relax the upper back and neck muscles.
2. Stretch the neck, shoulders, and upper back gently while the muscles are warm and pliable.
3. Finish with two minutes of ice to the most intense spot of pain in the neck and upper back to calm any inflammation that may have worsened with the heat.

Chapter 16: HERBAL REMEDIES AND THERAPEUTIC OILS FOR NECK PAIN

YOU'VE TRIED ALL OF THE TECHNIQUES mentioned in this book to treat your neck pain and relax, yet you still have pain that you cannot get rid of. You'd really like to take a pain pill, but you know you shouldn't. Instead, try some herbal alternatives. This chapter lists the herbal remedies and therapeutic oils that I have found to be helpful. You can find these at most health food stores, but I recommend asking your healthcare provider what brand they prefer (quality of brands changes over time).

White Willow Bark for Pain

White willow bark is the natural version of aspirin. Pharmacological companies discovered the active ingredient in white willow bark that decreased pain, and now they chemically produce it in a concentrated form. If aspirin were developed today, it would be labeled as a prescription drug because its lethal dose is so minuscule.

White willow bark contains aspirin in its natural state and is less likely to irritate the stomach lining or cause death. It is more expensive than a bottle of aspirin, but if you adhere to the lifestyle changes this book suggests, you should not need much of this herbal remedy.

Valerian Root for Better Sleep

Valerian root is a natural sleep aid. If you have difficulty sleeping, which can negatively affect your neck pain, valerian root may help. You can find it in pill form.

Kava Kava Root for Muscle Tension

Kava kava root is a natural muscle relaxer. It may help take the edge off neck pain caused by tense muscles.

Passion Flower for Relaxation

Passion flower can help you relax when you are feeling stressed or anxious, which can contribute to muscle tension. You can take it in the form of a tea, or for a stronger dose, you can take it as a tincture.

Caution!

As with any muscle relaxer or sleep aid, you should first try these remedies when you don't have to drive, work, or do anything that you would not do while impaired. It is best to take these herbs at night to help you relax and sleep.

Other Herbs That May Help

Other herbs that may help with your neck pain are, curcumin (a natural anti-inflammatory from turmeric that is best absorbed with pepper) and bromelain (a pineapple enzyme, another natural anti-inflammatory). I would not advise using these herbs without guidance from a practitioner who is well versed in herbal remedies.

Therapeutic Oils That May Help

Essential Oil of Peppermint for Muscle Aches

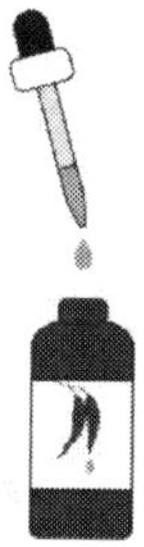

Essential oil of peppermint is good for tense muscles. It has a nice cooling effect, which also helps diminish muscle aches. Massage three to four drops of peppermint oil into the neck.

Essential Oil of Clove for Muscle Tension

Essential oil of clove is also good for muscle tension. Clove has a nice warming effect, which helps relax tense muscles. Massage three to four drops of clove oil into the neck and upper back.

Essential Oil of Lavender for Relaxation

Essential oil of lavender is a calming oil. Massage three to four drops of lavender oil into the chest. Combine this with some deep-breathing techniques, and feel your stress melt away.

Essential Oil of Marjoram for Increased Blood Flow

Essential oil of marjoram opens up blood flow, which helps facilitate healing. Massage three drops into the area of the body where you are experiencing the most tension (the front pectoral muscles, the upper back muscles, and/or the shoulders).

Essential Oil of Cypress for Edema

Essential oil of cypress reduces swelling, which can cause pain and limit healing. Massage a drop or two of cypress oil onto the regions that are swollen (the neck muscles, back, shoulders, and/or elbows).

My Advice on Using Natural Remedies

You can seek advice from a naturopath or another health practitioner who is well versed in herbs to find out if other herbal remedies would be better for your specific needs. However, like prescription medication, I am not a fan of relying on a surplus of pills, tinctures, etc. Natural or not, such treatments should be used sparingly so they work when you need them.

This is why it is important to have good practitioners on your healing team. It takes a village to help you obtain your optimal wellness!

Chapter 17: VITAMINS, MINERALS, AND SUPPLEMENTS FOR YOUR NECK PAIN

IF YOU ARE EXPERIENCING neck pain, it may be due (or at least partially affected by) a deficiency in a vitamin or mineral.

There has been much debate over whether people should take vitamins. If you are eating a healthy, varied, and whole-foods diet, you should be able to get all of your needed vitamins through your food. Unfortunately, most of our food is grown on over-farmed land, so the food produced on it is deficient of micronutrients and genetically designed to look good and have a longer shelf life (with no effect to its nutritional content or taste).

My general advice is to take a half dose of a multivitamin every day or two. That way you are less likely to be deficient in anything and you avoid the risk of overdosing on anything.

If you are taking a multivitamin, make sure the vitamins are coming from a plant source. Plants build vitamins via complex biochemical processes, producing one specific biomolecule. When vitamins are produced in a lab, an unnatural form can be produced and included in the multivitamin pill.

Calcium/Magnesium/Vitamin D Blend

Your muscles need calcium and magnesium to relax. If you are deficient in these minerals, you will experience muscle cramping. Taking this blend may help your neck muscles relax. Marrying it with vitamin D helps the absorption of calcium and magnesium.

Don't take calcium at the same time you take your multivitamin because it limits the absorption of some minerals like iron. I frown on multivitamins that tout different formulas, claiming a certain formulation is specifically for postmenopausal women because it has more calcium than other vitamins. Well, guess what? You are voiding most of that calcium out the other end.

I recommend that you take a small dose of a multivitamin in the morning and your calcium at night. That way you benefit from its muscle-relaxing properties before you go to bed. It may help you relax enough to aid in your ability to fall asleep and stay asleep. This property of calcium led to the old wives' remedy of drinking a warm glass of milk before going to bed to help you fall asleep.

Glucosamine Sulfate

Glucosamine sulfate works by supplying your body with the building blocks it needs to repair joints. It is not medicinal in that it doesn't block pain, so if your pain decreases, it is because your joints are healing!

If you want to see if glucosamine sulfate will help your neck pain, take at least 2,000 mg of it in three doses of 700 mg tablets (one dose with each meal). Follow this dosage for at least a month. If you feel better, try weaning down to one dose a day. If your pain returns, you will know you need a full dose to benefit from the supplement. Most people can maintain with 500 mg to 1,000 mg a day, but need at least 2,000 mg a day at the beginning.

Before you buy a bottle of glucosamine sulfate, you have to read the label. Some bottles say on the front label that they contain glucosamine sulfate for joint health, but when you look at the ingredient label, you find out that the tablets have glucosamine chondroitin with MSM (which has sulfur in it). It's like saying to someone, "Here is some water," and then giving them a container of hydrogen and another of oxygen. You can make water from it, but it is not water. So remember that glucosamine sulfate is not the same as glucosamine chondroitin and MSM.

Vitamin C

If your neck pain is from the delayed onset of muscle soreness after a workout, try taking extra vitamin C for a couple of days to help speed up the breakdown of metabolic waste from the overused muscles. Vitamin C also speeds healing by keeping blood vessels healthy. I will often take 1,000 mg or more of vitamin C daily for three days before doing something physically taxing (like going for a hike up a mountain over a weekend). Vitamin C is water soluble, so it is difficult (but not impossible) to overdose on, as long as you are drinking plenty of water and have healthy organs.

Vitamin B Complex

Your body needs vitamin Bs to make hormones (which help combat stress), to produce red blood cells (which bring oxygen to your muscles), and to maintain nerve function (which keep pain down and healing up). Vitamin B is also water soluble.

Drink Plenty of Water

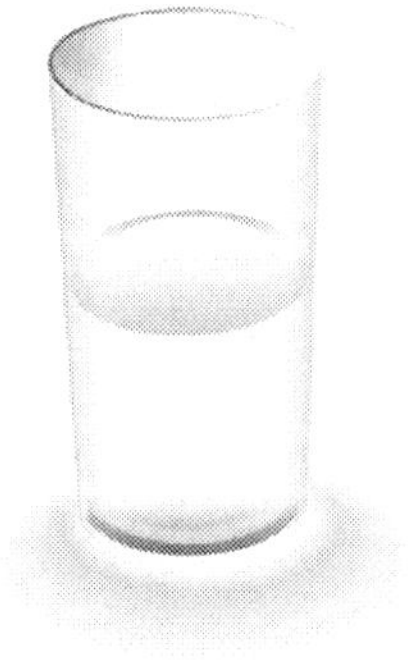

All tissues in our body need water. Dehydration affects blood pressure, muscle tension, and joint and fascia lubrication, all of which can lead to neck pain. (Fascia is the lining that covers muscles and organs in your body, separating the different tissues while holding everything together.)

You can calculate how much water to drink by multiplying your body weight by 2/3 (0.66). The result is the number of ounces of water you should drink in a day. For example, I weigh about 125 pounds, so I should drink approximately 83 ounces a day (125 x 2/3 = 82.5). Now, for every half hour you exercise, you should add at least 11 ounces. This is why I try to drink at least 96 ounces (three 32-ounce containers) of water a day.

If you drink black tea, coffee, and/or alcohol, you need to drink even more water. These beverages dehydrate you because they tamper with your anti-diuretic hormone (ADH). The hypothalamus (a part of your brain) detects how much water is in the blood. If the water content is low, the blood has a higher salt content. The pituitary gland (your body's master gland, also in the brain) senses this and releases ADH into the bloodstream. When the ADH reaches the kidneys, it opens the kidneys tubules so more water is reabsorbed into your blood instead of being urinated out (Figure 17-1).

After the water pressure goes back up, the hypothalamus detects this and tells the pituitary gland to stop producing ADH. The ADH in the blood drops, and the tubules in the kidneys close so more of the fluid will flow out into the urine. This negative feedback loop ensures that our blood holds the perfect amount of water.

If you drink too much water, the body has a means to urinate out the excess but keep a healthy amount in. As long as you have healthy kidneys and urinate when needed, it is almost impossible to overdose on water, but it's easy to be deficient in water. So drink up!

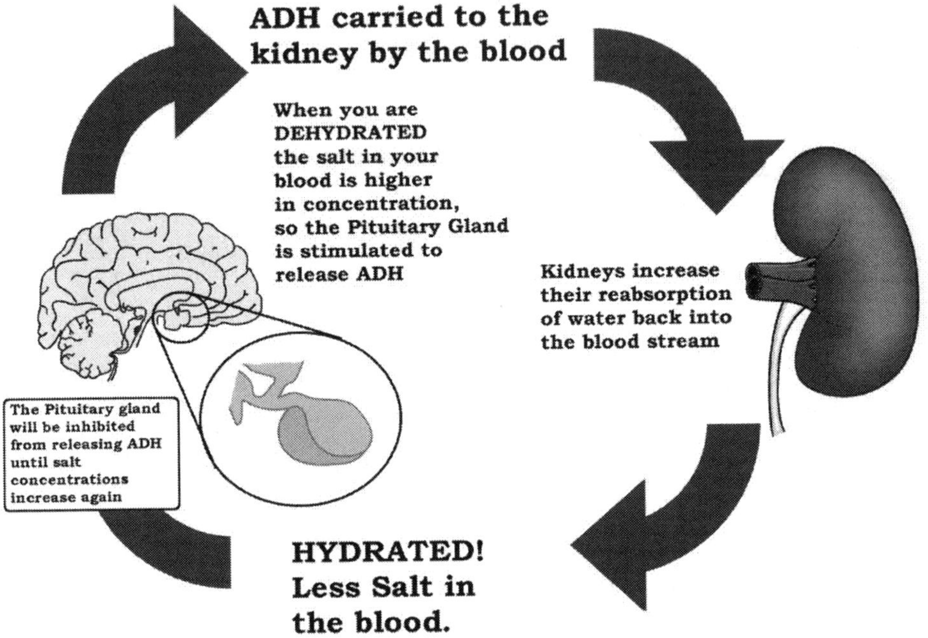

Figure 17-1: How the body regulates water.

When you drink tea, coffee, soda pop, or alcohol, ADH production goes down. This interferes with the regulation of water in the body, causing you to urinate out too much water. This leads to dehydration, which affects your health (especially over the long term). So for every ounce of alcohol and for every cup of tea or coffee you consume, you should drink at least 8 additional ounces of water.

Chapter 18: DEVICES THAT MAY HELP WITH YOUR NECK PAIN

IF YOU HAVE NECK PAIN, the following devices may help you alleviate it so you do not have to resort to taking pain medications.

TENS Unit

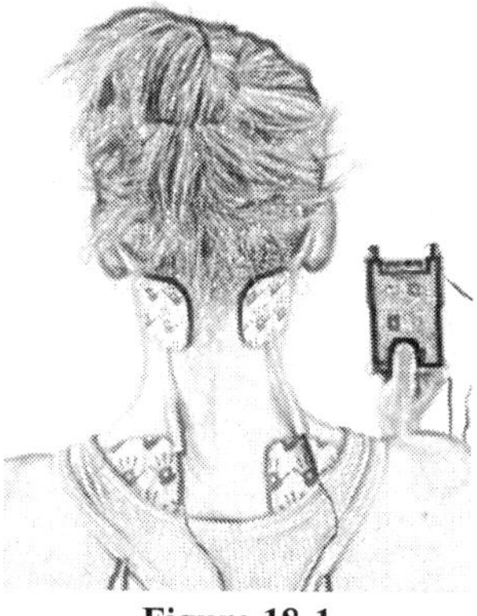

Figure 18-1

A TENS unit is a portable electrical stimulation unit that a patient can wear all day. It consists of a small electrical unit attached to electrodes in the form of sticky pads. You place the electrodes around the body part that hurts (at least a pad width apart). Figure 18-1 illustrates placement of the pads for tension neck pain: on the neck and at the base of the skull.

The electrical signals from the electrodes close the pain gates, diminishing the pain signals that are sent to the brain, and you feel the electrical pulse over the sensation of the pain. This is a passive, palliative treatment. I like these as an alternative to taking pain relievers because TENS units are very safe (the risks are nothing compared to pain pills).

TENS units are available at drugstores and online for less than $100. After the initial cost of the unit, you just need to replace the batteries and the sticky pads (they lose their stick after multiple uses).

Professional Massage Tools

If you suffer from neck pain, massage therapy is another treatment to consider. I prefer a professional massage from licensed massage therapists or healthcare providers like chiropractors and physical therapists.

Having muscle work performed by a healthcare provider, in my opinion, is even better than getting a massage from a massage therapist. Chiropractors and physical therapists have more knowledge of your condition, so they should be more effective at treating your condition.

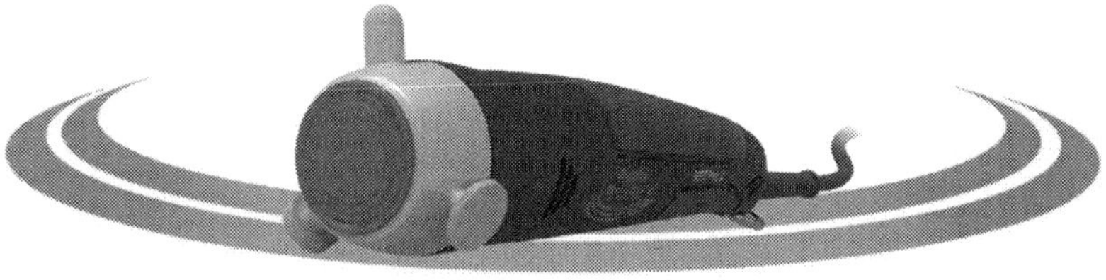

Figure 18-2: Rapid Release Technology (RRT).

I like to use the Rapid Release Technology (RRT; Figure 18-2) when I give my patients massages. The RRT uses painless, high-speed vibrations to melt scar tissue or adhesions found in spastic muscles and tender fascia.

When your body heals itself, it forms adhesions. Adhesions are stiff, ropey fibers that pull on healthy tissues. They can also impair blood flow and lymphatic drainage and pinch nerves. Because adhesions seriously impair the body's ability to function well, they must be broken up.

I prefer using the RRT because it feels good and doesn't hurt, compared with the pounding action of slower devices or the scraping action of contoured tools.

You can purchase the RRT online. I have had patients buy their own RRT so they could treat themselves more frequently in the comfort of their own home. The cost is high (about $1,500), but if you use the RRT thirty times, the cost comes to $50 per treatment. It more than pays for itself, because each time you use it the treatment is free.

You can check it out at:
https://rapidreleasetech.com/product/

Kinesio Tape for Neck Pain

Kinesio tape is a short, flexible cloth tape that is worn to relieve muscle pain or to encourage muscles to work more efficiently (Figure 18-3). Kinesio tape helps massage muscles as they move. With the proper application, the tape stretches and compresses, then relaxes with the body's movement, lowering the pressure. This pumping action aids in blood flow and lymphatic drainage, which facilitates healing.

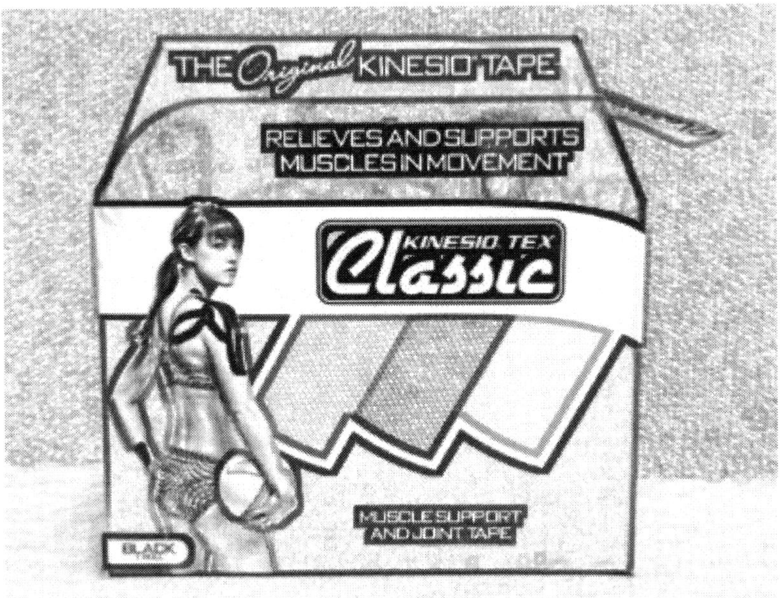

Figure 18-3: Kinesio tape.

It can also aid in the alignment of the body while it is in motion; for example, it can be applied to tug on the shoulders when they begin to slouch.

Kinesio tape has helped me as well as many of my patients

reduce pain. Some people claim kinesio tape only works because of the placebo effect. I say even if this is the only reason why it works, I will take a placebo over a toxic chemical any day, as long as it works without harm.[5]

Kinesio tape does no harm, is not expensive, and usually helps. This is why, despite the lack of strong scientific support, I have enough clinical "anecdotal" evidence to use it in my clinic.

Saunders Cervical Traction Unit

If your neck pain is due to nerve irritation from herniation(s) in your neck, a home traction unit may be a good idea (Figure 18-3). Explore the possibility with your healthcare provider.

My favorite home traction unit for the neck is the Saunders Cervical Home Traction Unit; the unit allows you to traction your neck at a specific poundage at an angle designed to open the space between the vertebrae in your neck. It is very effective at decompressing cervical discs; so much so, many suppliers require a prescription from a healthcare provider.

You can find new units selling for less than $400 online.

---

[5] Williams et al., "Kinesio Taping," *Sports Medicine.*

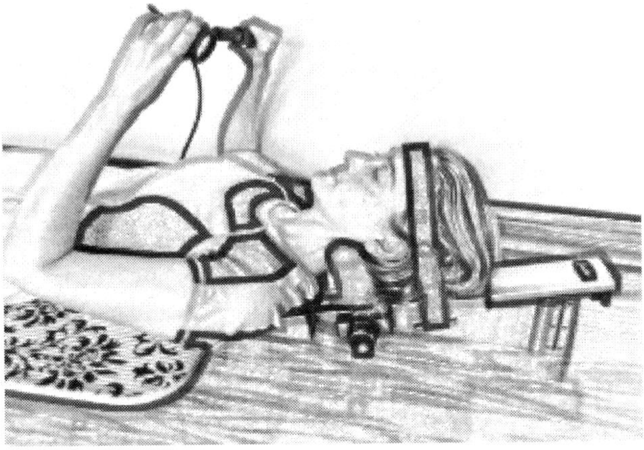

Figure 18-4: Using a home traction unit to relieve neck pain.

Yoga Trapeze

If your neck pain is due to nerve irritation from herniation(s) in your neck, another way to traction your neck is through inversions like handstands. For many, this is not possible, but maybe setting up a yoga trapeze in your home is.

First, confirm with your healthcare provider that this is a viable option for you. If it is, the trapezes are usually under $100. One inhibiting factor is the setup. You need to make sure that the trapeze is either tied or bolted securely onto beams that can bear the weight required.

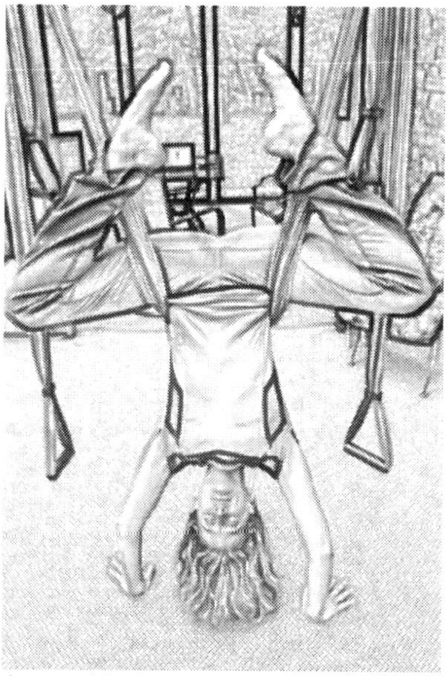

Figure 18-5: Hanging upside down on the yoga trapeze provides a couple of different ways to stretch the neck.

I set one up on my porch. I like the yoga trapeze because it makes inversions and stretching fun (unlike laying supine strapped into a contraption). So, whenever possible, I passively invert on the yoga trapeze, allowing the weight of my head to stretch out my neck (Figure 18-5).

Take a Yoga Class

Yoga is a great way to loosen tight muscles and joints, and it can help with neck pain if done correctly. However, as with any type of workout, it is possible to harm your body when doing yoga.

If you are naturally flexible, be especially careful with yoga. Most instructors are used to helping overly tight students, and

I have found that naturally flexible people are the most likely to be harmed by yoga because they tend to go too deep into a pose. Strengthening classes like Pilates tend to be more beneficial for such patients.

Regardless of what class you take, make sure you find a good instructor who can cater to your needs, modify poses to accommodate your condition, and keep it fun.

Start with a class with just a few other students so the instructor can give you more individual attention. Let the instructor know you are new. I prefer instructors who lay their hands on the attendees to assist them in correctly getting into a pose and using the correct muscle groups. A good instructor will also pay attention to the specific limitations of your body and modify the poses as necessary.

My general advice for people who suffer from neck pain is to attempt the exercises and stretches at 60 percent of your perceived ability. Over time, your 60 percent will be what your 100 percent would have been when you first started. If you are straining, you are likely straining your back, so *stop*.

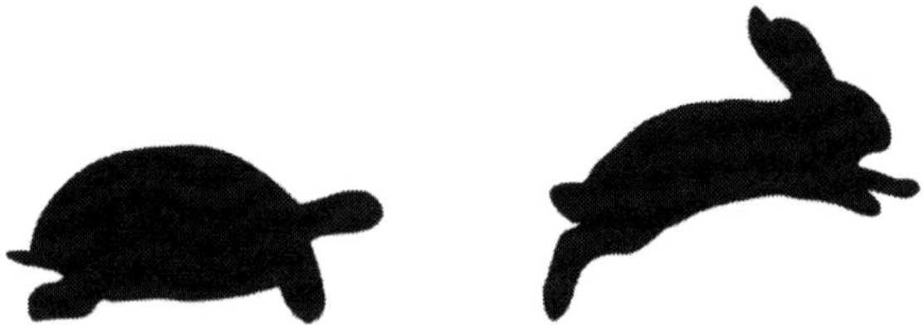

If you hurt yourself, you will not be able to continue with the exercise while you heal, and you may even backslide; it only takes seven days for muscles to atrophy, let alone weaken. If you go too fast from the beginning, you may have to start all over as the result of an injury, taking more time to reach your goal in the long run. Slow and steady wins the race.

Mouth Splint

If you have neck pain from jaw dysfunction, talk to your dentist to see if wearing a splint at night is a good option for you. At a minimum, wearing a mouth splint will protect your teeth if you grind your teeth at night. Bonus if it helps your neck pain.

If you suffer from jaw pain, clicking, or signs of jaw dysfunction (TMD), check out my book *Combat Jaw Pain.*

***

As in my other books, in these last few chapters, I talk about how chiropractic can help with neck pain, how it is safe, and how to find a practitioner who meets your needs. If you have read any of my previous books, this will be review.

I included my chapter on acupuncture, written with the help of my good friend and nationally known acupuncturist, Jennifer Stone, BS, LAc.

I have my chapters on Gua Sha and cupping as well, as these are also great techniques for neck pain.

If you have read these chapters before and choose not to reread these last chapters, let me say thank you for reading this book. I hope it helps you with your neck pain!

If you like this book, please let me know by writing a review on **Amazon**.

Thank you!

Chapter 19: WHY SEE A CHIROPRACTOR FOR YOUR NECK PAIN

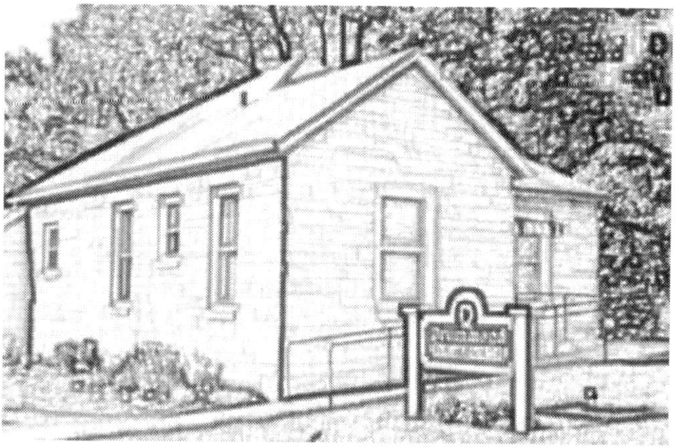

Figure 19-1: Dr. Karin's office.

SOME PEOPLE CONTEND THAT chiropractic medicine is less valid or less advanced than other forms of medicine. This is not true.[6] It is sad to me that many people still consider chiropractic an "alternative" medicine or think that chiropractors just treat neck or back pain.

---

[6] Bryans et al., "Evidence-based Guidelines for the Chiropractic Treatment of Adults with Headache," *Journal of Manipulative and Physiological Therapeutics*; Astin and Ernst, "The Effectiveness of Spinal Manipulation," *Cephalalgia*.

Chiropractors are primary care physicians who have as many years of education as a medical doctor. It only takes months to learn how to adjust, but years to learn differential diagnosis. A chiropractor knows when not to manipulate, when to refer a patient to someone else, and which specialist the patient should be referred to, if need be.

There is little mystery on why chiropractic works. It has been scientifically studied for its efficacy and economy for decades. Chiropractors are more than just neck and back doctors. They can help with so much more.

Chiropractors have more education in nutrition, anatomy, differential diagnostics, and imaging than medical doctors do. A medical doctor's education is filled with pharmacology, which chiropractors study minimally.[7]

Medication versus Chiropractic

When you seek medical treatment, a medical doctor typically treats you with a drug, whereas a chiropractor can help you find a way to heal without using medication to mute your symptoms.

There is a reason medications require a prescription. I have had many patients who suffered terribly after taking just a few doses of a new medication prescribed by their doctor. Some of their more common side effects have included chronic pain, hormone imbalance, weight gain, and depression.

---

7 Jensen, "Chiropractic Education vs. Medical Education."

Serious negative side effects are real and do occur. This is why I strongly believe that if you have the time to see if the natural route works for you, you should pursue it. Medicine is better suited for critical ailments when you do not have the time to allow your body to heal itself. To use medicine for anything else is unhealthy in the long run.

If you can get better with chiropractic treatment and lifestyle changes, those approaches are better than turning to a pain pill. If you go the prescription route for pain, you are not solving the problem. You're masking it and allowing the pain to worsen with time while the pain medication's efficacy wanes.

Starting with Chiropractic

If you suffer from neck pain, chiropractors can help you determine the cause of it. They will treat you and/or refer you to another healthcare practitioner if necessary. They can also teach you how to naturally alleviate neck pain.

I look forward to a time when patients try chiropractic first to see if it can help (knowing their chiropractor will send them to a medical doctor or surgeon if they feel the patient's condition is beyond what chiropractic can alleviate). Even if chiropractic does not work for you, you can always fall back on the medical route. But if you start with the medical route, especially surgery, sometimes there is no turning back.

I believe if people saw a chiropractor before going to a medical doctor, it would solve a lot of our healthcare problems in America (both the costs of healthcare and the general health of this country).

I love that I am married to a chiropractor. He can help keep my spine flexible and youthful. My goal is to feel well until I am at least 102 years old. I would say 120 years old, since some studies suggest that humans are genetically designed to live that long,[8] but we live on a polluted planet and I am not perfect…which is a good thing. Attempting to be perfect is too stressful, and stress leads to dis-ease, which leads to disease and early death.

---

[8] Ruiz-Torres and Beier, "On Maximum Human Life Span," *Advances in Gerontology*.

Chapter 20: CHIROPRACTIC MANIPULATION: WHAT IS IT, HOW CAN IT HELP, AND IS IT SAFE?

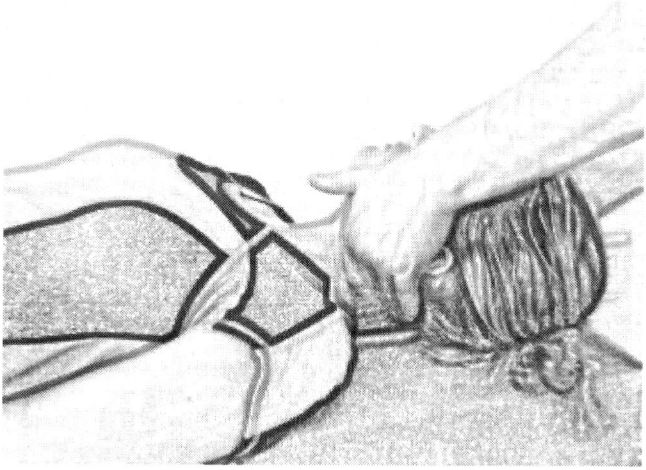

Figure 20-1

I MAY BE BIASED, but I believe that chiropractic manipulation to the cervical spine, the thoracic spine, and the cranial bones are the best treatments for most types of neck pain (Figure 20-1). I also believe people should have their low back and pelvis adjusted as well; if the pelvis is crooked, how can you expect the neck to stay straight? The whole spine sits on the pelvis. Remember, the eyes like to be level with the horizon, so if the base is crooked, the neck will have to tilt the opposite way for the eyes to be level.

I say, try chiropractic, especially since it is super safe and relatively affordable! It also often results in more health benefits than expected. Bonus! In this chapter, I explain the how and why. I hope this information encourages you to try chiropractic if you haven't already.

What Is a Chiropractic Manipulation?

During a chiropractic manipulation (also called an adjustment), a chiropractor applies a high-velocity, short-lever arm thrust to a bone to decompress a joint, restoring normal motion to the joint and/or normal alignment of the bones. Let me explain in layman's terms how a chiropractor does an adjustment.

To perform an adjustment, the chiropractor introduces a quick stretch to the muscles surrounding a joint while staying within the joint's normal range of motion.

Muscles have a quick stretch reflex, and when a muscle is stretched quickly, nerves in the muscle respond by causing the muscle to relax. This autonomic reflex protects the muscles from tearing during any quick stretch.

A chiropractic adjustment does not go nearly deep enough to risk tearing muscles, but the nerves and muscles do not know this. All they know is that an external force is making the muscles stretch quickly, so the nerves protect the muscle from such external forces. Therefore, an adjustment causes muscles to relax.

Fluid is present in the space between the bones. When a chiropractor performs a quick stretch, the barometric pressure on the joint fluid decreases (Figure 20-2). As with any fluid, decreasing the pressure releases gasses (in this case, oxygen, nitrogen, and carbon dioxide).

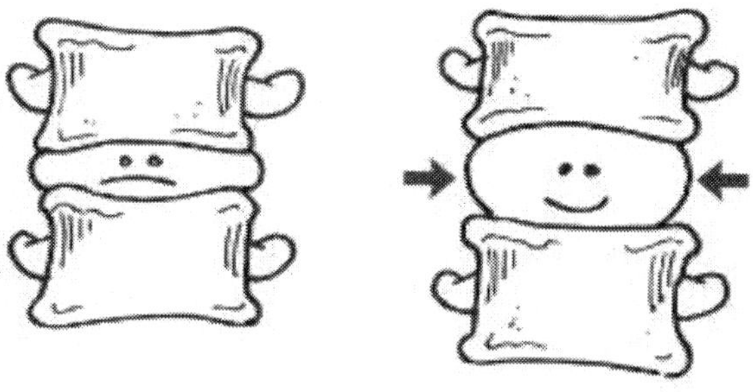

Figure 20-2: Releasing the pressure on joint fluid.

An everyday example of this phenomenon is when you open a can of soda. The soda in the can is under pressure, and when you open it, the pressure on the fluid decreases, and bubbles come out of the liquid. A joint, however, is a closed "container," so the "bubble(s)" pop immediately.

Why an Adjustment Helps

Many physiological events occur during an adjustment to facilitate healing. Examples of these amazing events are:

Increases Range of Motion

During an adjustment, a chiropractor moves a joint within its full healthy range of motion. It is safe because the chiropractor is far from overstretching the ligaments. If you do not move enough, your joints degenerate. When is the last time you stretched all of your joints to their full range of motion? There is a reason we say, "If you don't use it, you lose it." People stiffen as they get older not because of their chronological age, but because of their lack of stretching over time. Look at yogis. There are 100-year-old yogis who are more flexible than average middle-aged Americans.

I like to say that chiropractic manipulations are like going to a partner yoga class, but with a skilled partner who knows how to get to the end range of all your joints quickly and safely. Chiropractic adjustment is like yoga with an "oomph."

Reverses Degeneration

Bones and joints are not rods of iron that rust with time. They are living tissue that degenerates with aberrant stressors over time. Everyday activities result in micro trauma to tissues. As you age, your ability to heal slows down, so your body begins to lose the healing battle.

When you are young, you heal rapidly because the joints are plump with nutrient-filled fluid, which is why you do not feel this micro trauma occurring. Over time, abnormal stressors of our modern lifestyle cause the joint fluid to slowly seep out, and the cells inside start to die. With less nutrient-filled fluid and fewer cells to repair the damage as we age, each of these injuries is felt more profoundly. You take longer to heal, and the micro traumas begin to accumulate. This results in degeneration and arthritic changes.

But movement can help heal this damage. It was once thought that cartilage in the joints just wears away with time. Now we know that cells (chondrocytes) inside each joint repair the cartilage. Unfortunately, most people cause damage faster than the few chondrocytes can fix it, resulting in degeneration.

We need movement to support the cell repair and to facilitate the flow of nutrients in and waste out required for the repair process. Why?

Blood delivers nutrients to the joints, but for the nutrients to seep into the joint fluid, the fluid has to stir. Movement stirs the joint fluid and allows blood in the capillary bed to deliver nutrients deeper inside the joint fluid. The cells inside the joints receive the nutrients they need for this rebuilding process. Thus, simply moving your joints helps them heal.

When you sit or stand still for too long, the weight of your body slowly squishes the fluid out of your joints (Figure 20-3). Your joints become deficient of the much-needed nutrients that would normally flow into a healthy, moving joint. If you sit too long, you literally starve your joints,

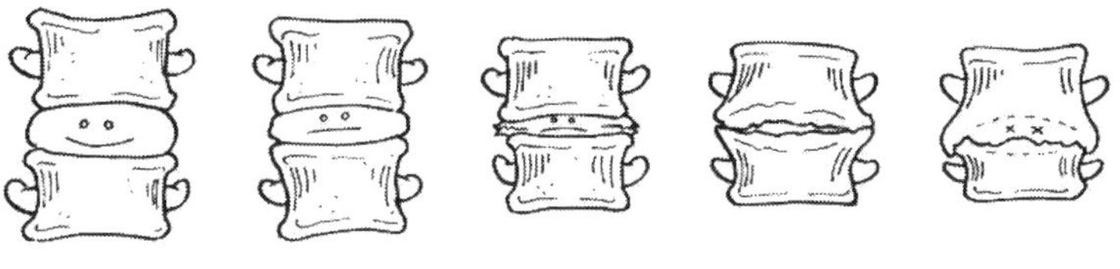

Figure 20-3: Discs degenerate over time because of a lack of movement.

causing them to degenerate over time.

Like physical movement, an adjustment literally "feeds" the joints it moves. When the gas bubbles form in the joint and pop, the fluid stirs (Figure 20-4). Nutrients flow in, facilitating the joint's healing and reversing the degenerative process.

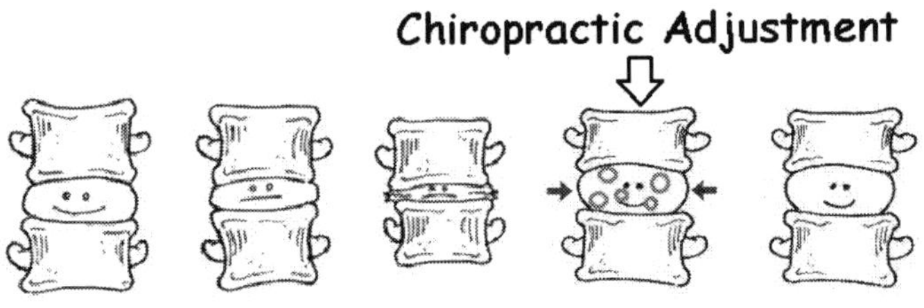

Figure 20-4: Chiropractic adjustment decompresses a joint, reversing the degenerative process.

The increased space between the bones takes the pressure off nerves (decreasing one's experience of pain) and allows for more blood flow and lymphatic drainage. All of this facilitates the healing of the surrounding tissues.

Even young adults who do not move enough will experience degeneration in their joints. I am seeing people at younger ages getting degenerative joint disease from sitting too much beginning early in their life.

Relaxes Spastic Muscles

An adjustment relaxes spastic muscles through the quick stretches I described earlier in the chapter.

This is why adjusting the neck (cervical spine) helps with neck pain. One quick adjustment relaxes the neck muscles far more effectively than a whole hour of massage. A cervical adjustment is far safer than taking pain medication in the long run, and it corrects the cause of neck pain, unlike pain medication, which just masks the pain.

Healing Occurs, Even at a Biochemical Level

During an adjustment, other biochemical reactions occur. The body releases endorphins into the area of the adjustment. This provides the short-term pain relief people report after an adjustment. The long-term effects of an adjustment are faster healing and restored full range of motion.

Chiropractic Adjustments Are Safe

I have patients who come in very concerned about getting their neck adjusted, even though, in my opinion, an adjustment is one of the best treatments for neck pain. Unfortunately, these patients have heard that neck adjustments can cause paralysis or strokes.

If a patient has paralysis or a stroke after seeing a chiropractor, then that patient was at risk of paralysis or stroke from any regular activities of daily living. An adjustment does not move the neck outside of the normal range of motion. For something terrible to go wrong, the neck had to have an abnormality that made the patient vulnerable with any kind of movement. Tilting the head back to wash their hair could cause as much injury.

Just by living you are at risk of having a stroke. I have adjusted the necks of several thousand patients dozens, if not hundreds, of times to date. That is tens, if not hundreds, of thousands of neck adjustments I have personally performed. Every one of my patients feels an increase of motion, and most feel an immediate relief of pain after a neck adjustment. Not one of my adjustments has resulted in a stroke, let alone paralysis.

In fact, you are just as likely to have an adverse vascular event within twenty-four hours of seeing your regular doctor as when seeing your chiropractor.[9] Either you are going to have a stroke or not. Sadly, if it happens after seeing a chiropractor, some people want to blame the chiropractor.

Even medical organizations can't deny that chiropractic adjustments are safe.[10]

You are more likely to be struck by lighting (1 per 0.96 million lightning strikes)[11] in any given year than to be seriously hurt by a manipulation to the neck (1 per 1.565 million manipulations).

Research validates that chiropractic manipulation is much safer than taking NSAIDs.[12] Yet people in our culture are

---

[9] Cassidy et al., "Risk of Vertebrobasilar Stroke and Chiropractic Care," *Spine.*

[10] Mayo Clinic, "Chiropractic Adjustment."

[11] National Weather Service, "How Dangerous is Lightning?"

[12] Blower et al., "Emergency Admissions for Upper Gastrointestinal Disease," *Alimentary Pharmacology and Therapeutics*;

generally more comfortable taking a pain pill than having a neck manipulation! I believe this is due to misinformation. In fact, people *die daily* due to medicine taken as prescribed. Yet most people feel comfortable taking their medications!

Even the Side Effects of Spinal Manipulation Are Often Beneficial

The health benefits of an adjustment are often greater than expected. By stretching the vertebrae of the spine apart and creating more space for the nerves that exit the spinal cord, blood flow and lymph drainage increase. This allows nutrients to flow into and waste to flow out of the tissues, resulting in ideal conditions for the tissues to not only heal, but to function optimally. Without this space, there is more pressure on the nerves, blood vessels, and tissues.

Nerves especially do not like pressure; they function better with space. Better communication between the brain and the body makes for better functioning organs, leading to a healthier body in general. This is why patients often report their neck pain resolves, their sinuses drain, the pressure in their ears clears, and they no longer suffer from headaches after a neck adjustment. These are all great side effects for those suffering from neck pain. This is why I love chiropractic.

Nerves that exit the neck region send signals to the head and upper extremities (Figure 20-5). If these nerves are being

---

Fries et al., "Toward an Epidemiology of Gastropathy," *Gastroenterology*.

compressed, they will cause head, neck, arm, or hand pain (Figure 20-6).

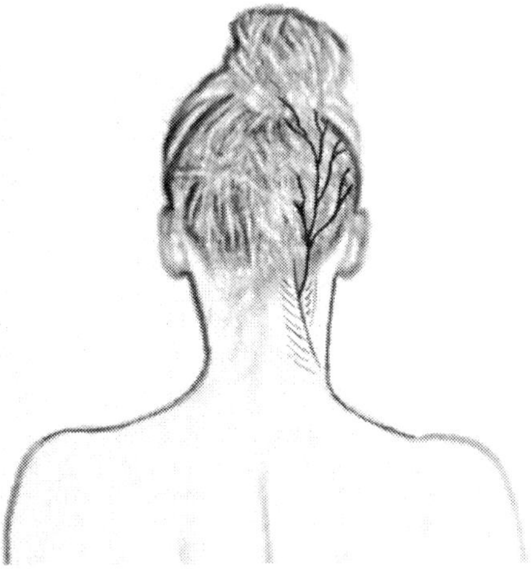

Figure 20-5: Neck adjustments take pressure off the nerves that exit the neck region, often providing relief from neck pain and headaches.

After treating neck pain with a cervical (neck) adjustment, I often hear things like "I haven't had a migraine since," "My sinuses have cleared," "My vertigo is gone," "My carpal tunnel syndrome resolved," and "My arms don't fall asleep or hurt anymore."

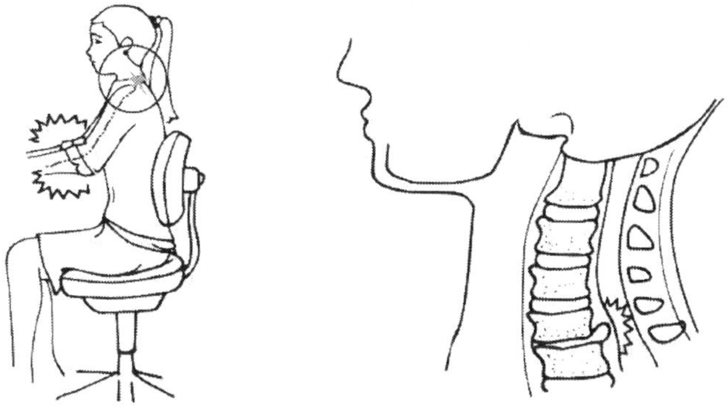

Figure 20-6: Example of a nerve being pinched in the neck, resulting in arm pain, numbness, tingling, and/or weakness. This is why adjusting the neck can help alleviate arm pain.

Nerves that exit the mid-back region send signals to the organs in the mid torso, including the lungs, stomach, spleen, and liver. After treating for mid-back pain, I have heard things like "My GERD has improved" and "My asthma is better."

Nerves that exit the lower back region of the spine send signals to the organs in the lower torso, including the lower intestines, reproductive organs, and lower extremities. After treating lower back pain, I often hear things like "My bowel movements have been more regular than ever," "My menstrual cycle is more normal," "My ED (erectile dysfunction) seems to have resolved," and "I was told by my medical doctor that I was infertile, and now I am pregnant!"

After treating children, their parents report, "They are calmer," "They are sleeping better," and "They are able to focus more."

I prefer these types of "side effects" to the side effects people experience with allopathic medicine, which often have incredibly long lists of possible negative side effects, including "Can cause death." When you take any medicine, there is always some negative effect; sometimes that negative effect ends up outweighing the benefit.

Finding Relief with Chiropractic after a Car Crash

I personally found relief from chiropractic adjustments after I was in a car crash in 2014. For the first week, I was in severe pain and could hardly move my neck. I was as stiff as a board.

A week of muscle therapy got me to the point where my husband, Dr. Dallas Drummond, and I felt like I could tolerate an adjustment (I desperately needed one).

We went to our office, and after a quick palpation of my neck, Dallas said he was sure I was still so tight because I simply needed a good, old-fashioned, rotary neck adjustment. Until then, all I could tolerate was my mid-back being adjusted and my neck being mobilized and massaged.

I have been adjusted thousands of times over my life, but that was the first time I honestly feared getting my neck adjusted. I now understand why some of my patients fear it.

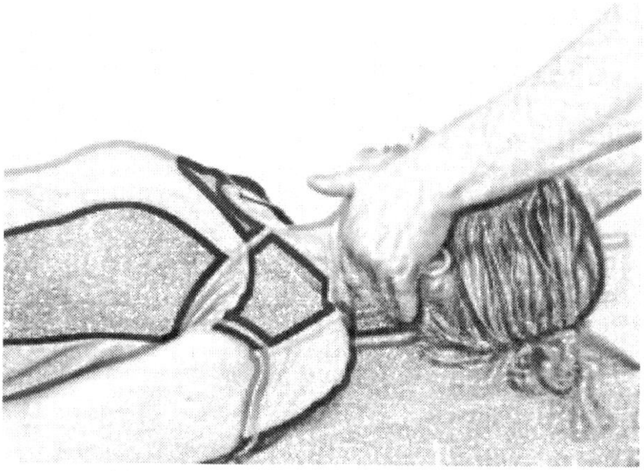

Figure 20-7: Getting my neck adjusted.

How could a fast thrust feel good on something that was super-sensitive to light touch? But my neck was not getting better with stretching and muscle work alone. I gave my husband the OK.

After a couple of quick twists and huge cavitations (popping sounds), I wanted to sing *hallelujah*! I could move my neck completely with minimal pain!

Relief!!!

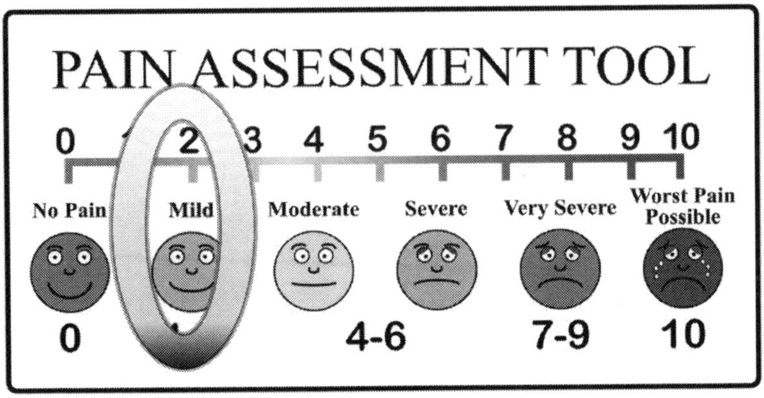

At the time, I had been a chiropractor for fourteen years but had never personally needed a spinal manipulation for such a severe physical ailment. Yes, I have woken up with a stiff neck a few times over the years and was spoiled by having a husband who I could nudge awake to get immediate relief. But this was the first time where I was in so much pain that I was afraid to get adjusted.

So when I felt immediate relief, my first thought was, "Holy cow! Adjustments really do work!"

Well, duh. I do this for a living and see it work several times an hour every workday. But to experience it firsthand like that made me understand on a whole new level why so many of my patients sigh with huge relief after an adjustment and often want to see me more frequently than I prescribe.

Because I was in that golden period of pain relief, I could lay on my stomach so Dallas could adjust the base of my neck in the prone position. Up until now, I couldn't lay on my stomach because it caused too much pain in my neck. But now I was ready to try it because I was in that 20-minute window when pain-relieving hormones were flooding through my neck muscles after the adjustment. I turned over and was able to rest my head on the headrest without feeling stabbing pain in my neck or back.

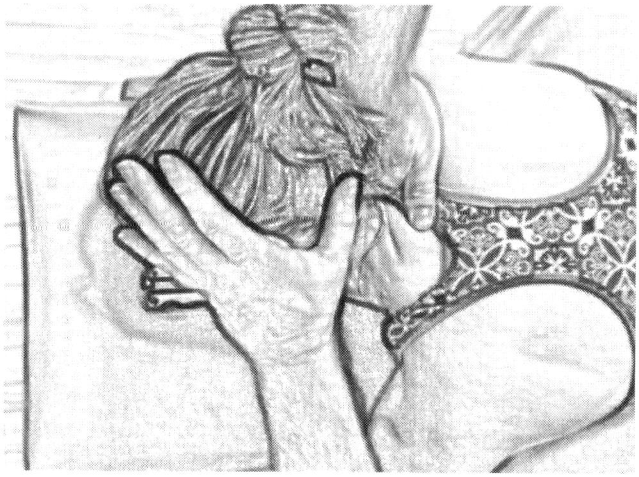

Figure 20-8: Dr. Dallas adjusting my C-T joint (the base of my neck where my cervical spine meets the thoracic spine)..

Dallas adjusted the base of my neck (Figure 20-8). I have no words to describe the sensation that coursed through my body. In a lame attempt, all I can suggest is that it was absolutely euphoric.

It was not the first time, nor the last time, I was super-glad to have married a chiropractor.

Determining Whether Neck Manipulation Is Right for You

I hope the information in this chapter has helped persuade you to see a chiropractor to determine if a neck adjustment is an appropriate treatment for your neck pain.

If you are going to receive a manipulation, simply ask how many manipulations your chiropractor performs on a weekly basis and how long they have been in practice. Ask how successful they are at treating neck pain like yours. The answers to these questions will help you figure out how skilled and practiced the chiropractor is at treating your condition.

I had a patient who had a seriously herniated disc in his neck. It was so severe that his left arm was going numb, his grip was weakening, and at best, he was in tremendous pain. I was worried I wouldn't be able to help him fast enough to avoid permanent nerve damage. I referred him to several surgeons, and the earliest he could be seen was in a week. I treated him three times during that week and showed him how to traction his neck in between visits. I was excited when he began showing more relief than I dared hope for, but I encouraged him to keep his appointment with the surgeon, who would order an MRI, just in case his condition worsened.

The surgeon, upon seeing his MRI, told my patient that he had no option but to have surgery and that chiropractic adjustments are very dangerous for his condition. The surgeon claimed if the man did not have surgery, he was going to have permanent nerve damage. The earliest the doctor could schedule the surgery was two weeks out.

Upon hearing this, I was shocked. I believed there was definitely hope of avoiding surgery because my patient was already showing signs of improvement. His grip was strengthening, he was rarely numb, but he was still in a lot of pain. I told the patient if he got all of his nerve symptoms resolved, he wouldn't need the surgery.

The patient was understandably very nervous to continue his chiropractic care because the surgeon had warned it would make his herniations worse, but because I had helped him so much already and he really did not like the idea of having his neck cut into, he figured it was worth a try.

Within two weeks, he was feeling well enough to cancel the surgery, and to this day, he is so grateful he gave me a chance. He still sees me once a month or so, mainly for low back issues because he sits too much. The last time I saw him, he said his neck continues to feel 100 percent.

If he didn't have a good relationship with a skilled chiropractor, he would have likely had the surgery. Once you are cut, there is no going back. Additionally, you are left with scar tissue, which limits your likelihood of getting back to 100 percent. Now, there are conditions in which you don't have time for manual therapies to assist your healing process, and I am grateful we have the option of surgery for these situations. But, in general, most neck issues don't need surgery.

This is another reason why it is important to have a team of healthcare professionals who can help you determine the treatment for your ailment. A surgeon is likely going to think you need surgery. A chiropractor is likely to think you need adjustments. An acupuncturist is likely to think you need acupuncture. So how do you go about finding good healthcare providers? I explain that in a later chapter. But first, let's look at what acupuncture can do for your neck pain.

Chapter 21: ACUPUNCTURE FOR NECK PAIN

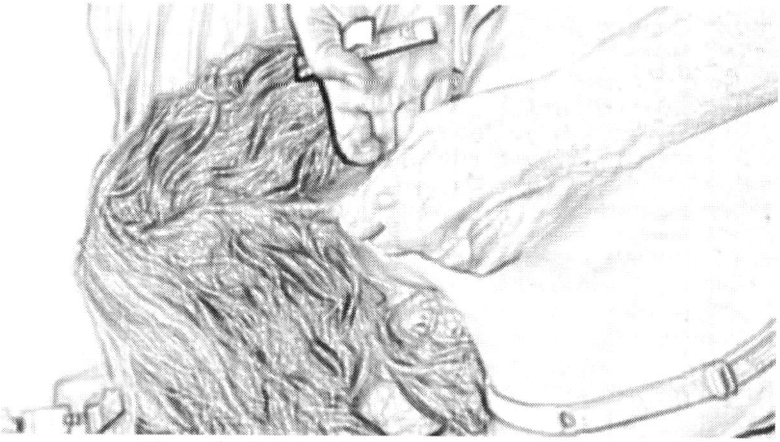

Figure 21-1: Receiving an acupuncture treatment.

YOU MAY BE hesitant to try acupuncture to treat your neck pain, or you may be fearful of having needles stuck into your muscles. I have a phobia of needles myself, yet acupuncture does not bother me. It helps that the needles are tiny and they do not inject or draw anything from my body. Most of the needles you barely feel. I will admit, some needles may go into a tender spot; if the area is too tender, you can have the practitioner remove the needle. You can always try that spot again at a future appointment. As your health improves, fewer and fewer spots should be tender.

If you find most of the needles uncomfortable, you can ask the practitioner to use smaller needles. After my whiplash injury from the car crash, I could barely handle the tiniest of needles. Some needles are so tiny that you should not be able to feel them at all. I knew I was improving as the needles became painless and I was able to use larger needles with each subsequent visit.

I encourage you to read the following Q&A with my acupuncturist to understand what acupuncture is and how it may be able to help.

Interview with Jennifer Stone, BS, LAc

When I decided to start seeing an acupuncturist, I chose Jennifer Stone, BS, LAc, because I had heard that she is not only a great acupuncturist, but a famous one! Her research has furthered her profession, and she has been an instructor for acupuncture.

Because many people are unfamiliar with acupuncture, I asked Jen to explain the procedure.

What is Acupuncture?

Acupuncture is a procedure in which fine needles are inserted into specific points on the body to relieve pain and promote homeostasis. Acupuncture originated in China and is the result of more than four thousand years of empirical evidence. Acupuncture has been shown to be an effective treatment for twenty-eight diseases, symptoms, or conditions.[13]

What Schooling/Licensure Is Required?

A licensed acupuncturist requires three years of post-graduate training for a master's degree and two additional years for a Doctor of Oriental Medicine degree.

Most states require NCCAOM (National Certification Commission for Acupuncture and Oriental Medicine) board certification to receive a license. Some states allow MDs and chiropractors to practice acupuncture with two hundred to three hundred hours of acupuncture training.

How Can it Help?

When an acupuncture needle is inserted into the skin, the body reacts, blood flow increases, and a variety of chemicals are released that reduce inflammation, stop pain, and promote healing.

---

13 World Health Organization, "Acupuncture: Review and Analysis"; Stone and Johnstone, "Mechanisms of Action for Acupuncture," *Current Treatment Options in Oncology*.

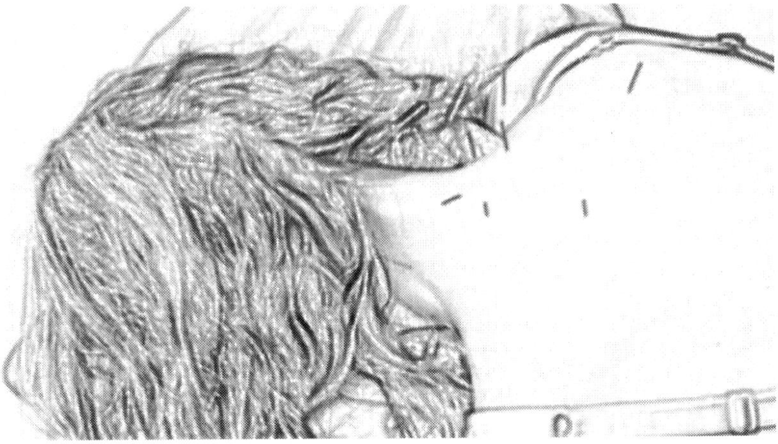

Figure 21-2: Acupuncture for the neck.

Are There Side Effects?

Sometimes patients have mild bruising or itching at the needle site. Occasionally someone will faint.

Are There Different Types of Acupuncture?

Yes. Traditional Chinese medicine (TCM), Japanese meridian style, auricular (ear) acupuncture, five element style, and Korean style are commonly practiced in the United States.

How Is Acupuncture Different than a Physical Therapist's Dry Needling?

There is no difference. Dry needling is acupuncture, and acupuncture needles are used. The company that began marketing dry needling training to physical therapists invented the term. The training is as little as twelve hours with no clean needle technique training and is not accredited.

Is Acupuncture Safe?

Yes. A recent review of acupuncture for low back pain reported that out of 7,161 people, no serious adverse events associated with the acupuncture were reported. Some cases of pneumothorax (lung collapse from puncture) have been reported in recent years, but all of them were caused by physical therapists who did not have sufficient training in acupuncture.

This last question brought up an important point. If you are going to try a treatment, be it acupuncture, chiropractic, or something else, make sure the practitioner is not only properly accredited, but has a good reputation. If a patient is hurt during a treatment, don't blame the tool or technique; instead, question the ability of the one yielding the tool or performing the technique.

Chapter 22: GUA SHA

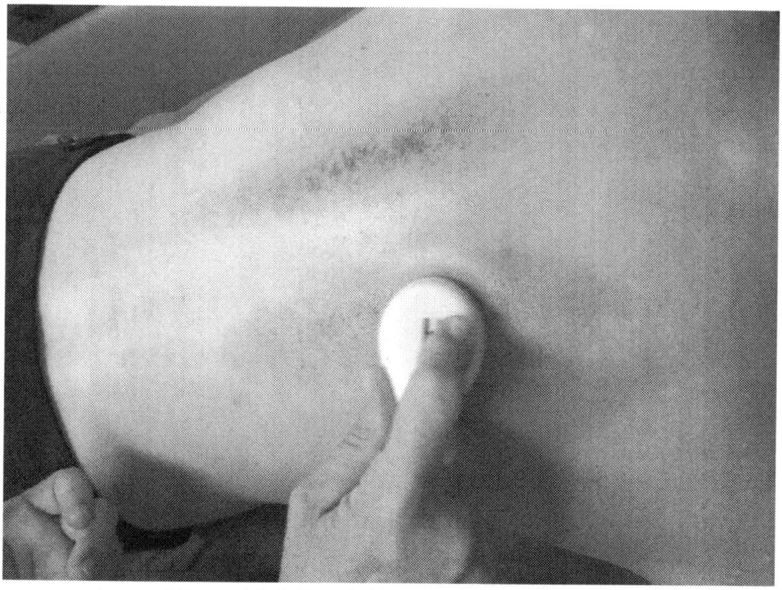

Figure 22-1: Receiving a Gua Sha treatment.

BEFORE I EXPLAIN Gua Sha, you need to know a little bit more about how your body works to better understand how this ancient Asian technique affects you.

Every cell naturally produces lactic acid as a waste product. Muscles and skin contain significant amounts of blood vessels that drain waste from and bring nutrients to their tissues. But the fascia (connective tissue) between the skin and muscles does not contain a lot of blood vessels. Lactic acid can build up in this layer and irritate the nerves, resulting in pain.

Introducing Gua Sha

Gua Sha is a treatment that releases the toxic lactic acid from the fascia, facilitating healing. The skin reddens (as shown in Figure 22-1), but this is not bruising because it does not turn blue (a bruise is full of blood that decreases in oxygen, turning it blue); the redness diminishes over two to five days (unlike a bruise which can take more than five days).

The Graston Technique is a new age technique based off Gua Sha. It has been heavily marketed as being effective at releasing lactic acid, but I find the Graston specialized tools are not worth the money. A soup spoon in a skilled hand such as my acupuncturist's, Jennifer Stone, BS, LAc, is just as good (if not better).

Gua Sha (and Graston), when done well, should not bruise the skin or tissue; it should only leave it reddened. If you are bruised by a treatment, it likely was done too roughly. Bruising is caused by damaging tissue, which does not facilitate healing. Again, you can tell if the procedure was effective (versus rough) by the length of time it takes the redness to disappear (which should be within a couple of days) and if it fades versus turning blue.

My Personal Story

After my motor vehicle crash, I was too tender to handle chiropractic manipulation or even acupuncture. After several weeks, I was relieved when my acupuncturist agreed that I was finally ready for a Gua Sha treatment. As she scraped the spoon along my paraspinal muscles (Figure 22-2), I felt a rope of tissue in my mid-back in the exact region I felt the most injured. This told me that my damaged tissues were tightening as they healed, forming unhealthy adhesions that could leave me vulnerable to future injuries and/or re-exacerbations.

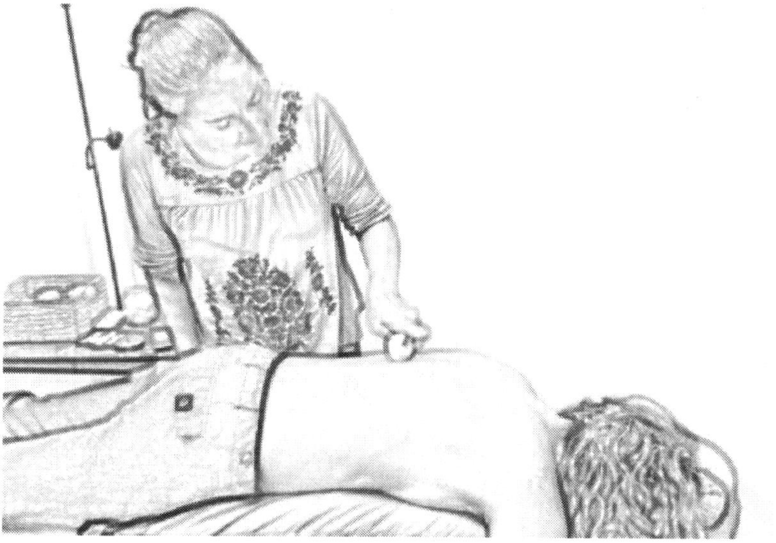

Figure 22-2: Jennifer Stone, BS, Lac, giving me a Gua Sha treatment.

The tissue was so tight that as she scraped over it, it tugged at my sides, feeling like it was pulling the periosteum (the membrane that lines the bones) off my ribs. She worked on it for a few more minutes, but the sensation didn't diminish. As bad as I was, it would take several sessions to work out that tissue. It did eventually work out, and I will be forever grateful that I was able to restore normal fluidity of my muscle movement.

If you attempt to work out when your muscles are adhering to your bones aberrantly (be it your chest wall or your neck), your condition can worsen as the muscles strain against these adhesions. Plus, these adhesions reduce the flow of blood in and waste out, making unfavorable conditions for regaining strength in your muscles.

Chapter 23: CUPPING FOR THE NECK

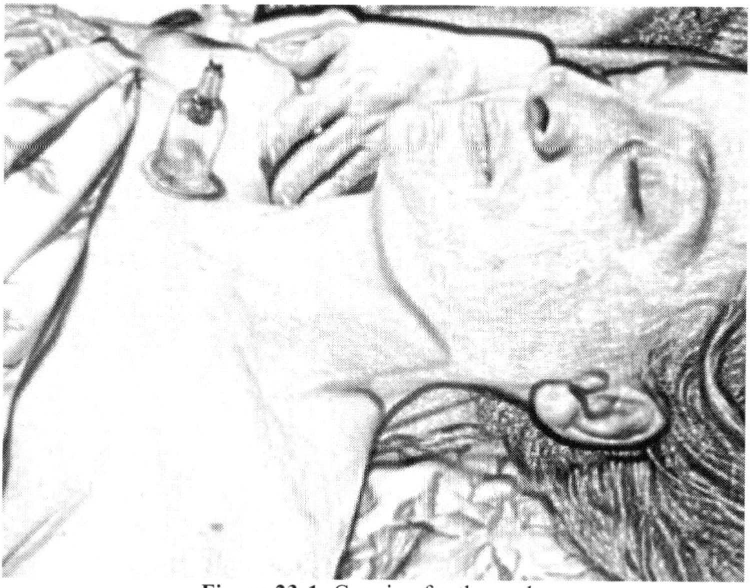

Figure 23-1: Cupping for the neck.

IF YOU'VE SEEN LARGE, perfectly round discolorations on an athlete's skin, you've seen the outward signs of cupping.

Cupping involves creating negative pressure on tissues. A therapist uses a cup to create a vacuum that draws the skin up and away from the muscles (Figure 23-1). This is the opposite of negative pressure used during a regular massage, where the practitioner physically presses on the tissue to push out the metabolic waste and break up adhesions.

There are a variety of ways to create negative pressure with cupping. Glass cups are usually used because they are durable and easy to sanitize. Different sized cups are used for different sized muscles and different applications (Figure 23-2).

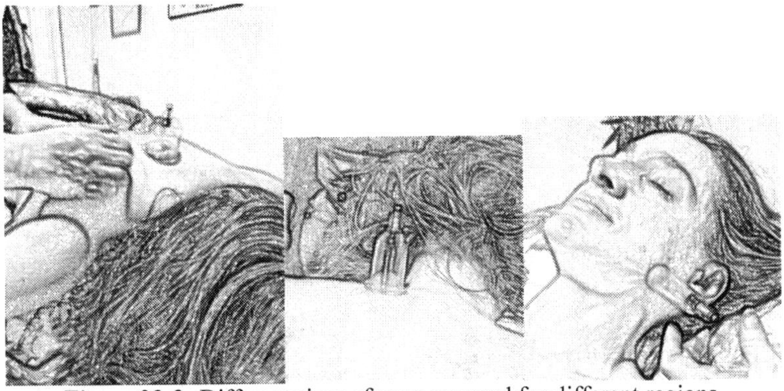

Figure 23-2: Different sizes of cups are used for different regions.

The vacuum in the cup can be created a variety of ways. One involves heating the air inside the glass cup and then placing it on a trigger point or acupressure point. As the air cools, it creates a vacuum, and the skin gets drawn up into the cup. A newer technique uses a pump to suck the air into the cup to create a vacuum, as shown in Figure 23-3.

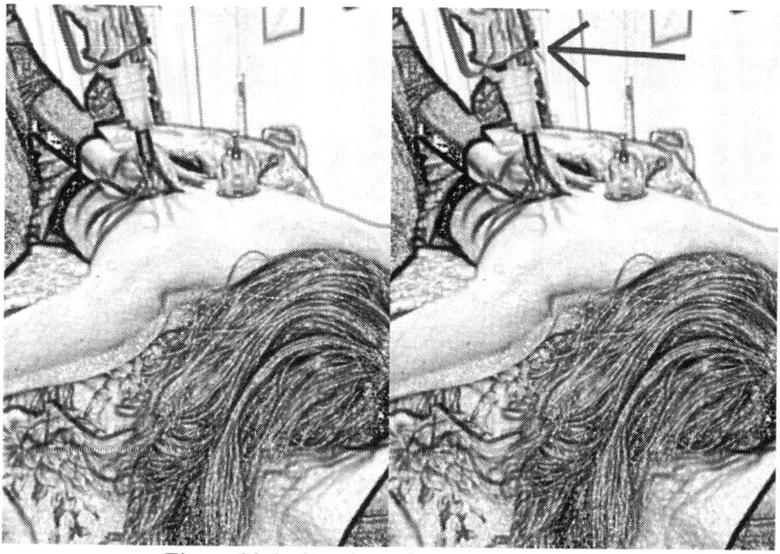

Figure 23-3: Cupping using a suctioning tool.

As the skin gets sucked into the cup (Figure 23-4), the skin layer separates from the muscle layer, breaking up adhesions in the fascia. Leaving the cup at these points for a few minutes brings more blood to these tissues. As a result, the tissues heal, and their function improves.

Leaving a cup on a spot for too long can cause bruising or blistering, so be sure to communicate to your practitioner if the cups are getting uncomfortable.

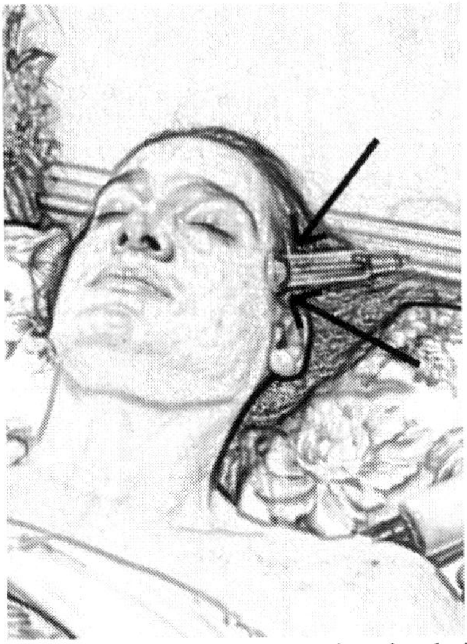

Figure 23-4: Showing the skin of the temporal region being sucked into the cup, bringing more blood to the region, facilitating healing.

A New Application for This Ancient Tool

Some massage therapists use cups as a massage tool. They apply oil to the skin first so they can glide the cup over a region (Figure 23-5). This type of massage is a negative pressure massage. Unlike a regular massage, in which positive pressure squishes metabolic waste out of the muscles, a massage therapist can use the negative pressure of the cup to milk metabolic waste out of the region by gliding the cup over a region.

You may prefer this negative massage to a deep-tissue (positive) massage when you are too tender to handle pressure to a tissue. Some find this technique more comfortable. Some prefer positive pressure. The only way to know which you prefer is to try each and decide for yourself which feels more comfortable and effective for you.

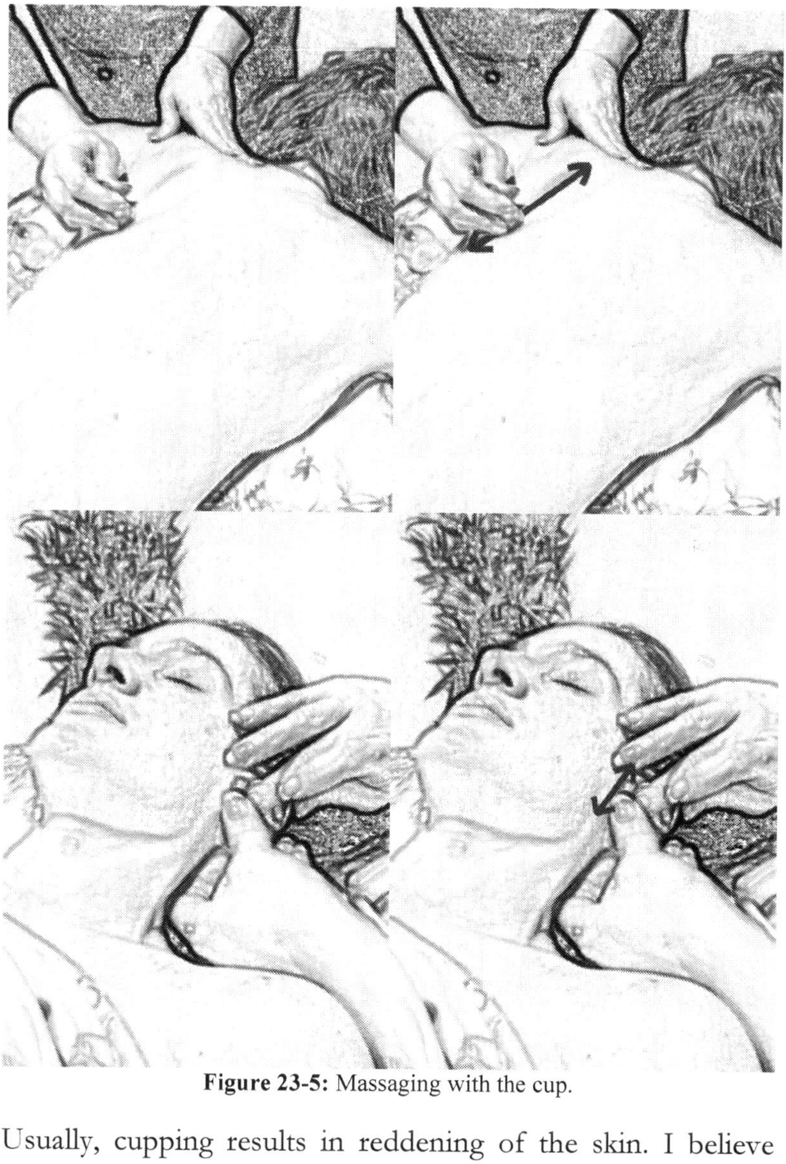

Figure 23-5: Massaging with the cup.

Usually, cupping results in reddening of the skin. I believe that if you bruise heavily afterwards, the practitioner used too much suction on you. More is not always better. Bruising is a sign of tissue damage, not healing, but sometimes a little bruising is unavoidable. When cupping is done well, bruising should be minimal, and the reddening of the skin should fade within a few days.

I have heard that when done well, cupping also helps with wrinkles because it brings blood to the surface, feeding the skin and keeping it plump. Bonus!

Chapter 24: WHAT TO LOOK FOR IN A PRACTITIONER

HOW DO YOU FIND a practitioner (be it a chiropractor, medical doctor, massage therapist, physical therapist, osteopath, naturopath, acupuncturist, or any other type of healer) or a group of healers to help you treat your neck pain? This is a loaded question, but the following are my two cents of advice.

First, find your practitioners by asking friends and family for referrals. The internet is a good place to find out more about a practitioner, but it is not the best place to choose one. Anyone can look good online and post fake testimonials. Try to use sites like www.yelp.com where people can post good and bad reviews without the business owners cherry-picking only the good reviews. This will increase the likelihood of getting legitimate evaluations.

Try to find people who have seen the specific practitioner you're considering and ask them about their experience.

Does the Practitioner Really Listen to Me?

Sadly, many in the medical field are in it for the wrong reason, or their reasons do not match your needs. You need to find a practitioner who has a passion for helping their patients. One indicator of this is how well they listen to their patients during an appointment. Most proper diagnoses come from taking an accurate history and getting a complete description of the current symptoms. Most physical examination, imaging, and laboratory work is performed to verify the diagnosis, not to find the problem.

Unfortunately, many doctors get burned out because of the fiasco that is the current political and insurance landscape. They are forced to see more people in less time and are required to complete more paperwork and coding of a patient's symptoms. Eventually, many practitioners end up shutting down emotionally, closing off their humanity in order to survive everything that's expected of them.

Doctors are people too, but you should not place the doctor's needs above your own when seeking treatment. Find a doctor whom you like on a personal level and who genuinely seems to care for you. This will positively affect your healing.

Does the Practitioner Give Me the Time I Need?

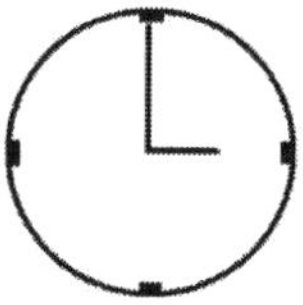

Understand that more time does not necessarily mean a greater quality of care. If the practitioner is efficient and very good, they will not need as much time, but you should feel like you received their full attention and a full treatment when you are with them. You should feel that you got what you needed. I always end my treatments by asking my patients if I took care of everything, or if there is something else they need. This assures me I covered what they came in for, and if I didn't, this gives the patient the opportunity to express their needs.

Sometimes I just need a few minutes to treat a patient; other times I end up spending a whole hour. It makes scheduling tough, but the rare times my patients have to wait, they know it wasn't because I overbooked but because someone needed more time. My patients appreciate that I give extra time if needed, and they recognize that someday it may be they who need that extra time.

Can the Practitioner Help Me? How Many Treatments Will it Take? How Much Will it Cost?

Ask the practitioner at the beginning whether your aliment is something they understand, have experience with, and have had success treating. What do they think your prognosis is? Will they be able to treat you within a reasonable budget?

If the treatment is costly, maybe you can find a less costly fix while still maintaining the quality of care. Costlier does not necessarily mean higher quality care. Beware, however, that you sometimes get what you pay for. Do not shortchange the quality of your healthcare to the point of negatively affecting your health.

If the practitioner does not think you have a good prognosis, don't waste your time or money on them! If your prognosis is bad, that is simply an opinion of someone who has not routinely seen success with your ailment. Find a different practitioner, one who has had success with your ailment, so they can give you a better prognosis.

For example, I have had patients who were told by several practitioners that they would never be able to turn their head fully left or right ever again because they had worn a neck collar for months after having broken bones in their neck. When you stabilize joints, such as by wearing a collar, you prevent movement. Like the old saying goes, "If you don't use it, you lose it."

Accordingly, when their doctors had them finally remove the collar, they ended up with an immobile, very stiff neck. Many of these post-neck-fracture patients completed a course of physical therapy, which helped loosen up the neck somewhat by stretching the muscles. Even so, these patients were still severely limited by the immobilized joints in the neck.

Some of these patients were told by their medical doctors never to try chiropractic. I find it interesting that a medical doctor who is not trained in a technique like chiropractic feels qualified to restrict a patient from choosing that treatment option. I would never tell a patient that they should not take a medicine; that is not in my scope of practice. With that said, I have had many allopathic doctors suggest chiropractic to their patients.

I have also had patients who were told by another chiropractor that they could not get an adjustment because they had a history of having a broken neck and their joint planes were no longer normal (because their bones healed aberrantly).

Thankfully, all of these people had friends or family members who knew me. Their friends or family members told them that they should at least consult with me, if for no other reason to get my opinion. I need only a few minutes to examine the neck to tell if I can help them or if I need to refer them to a specialist.

My goal with these cases is to see within six visits some improvement in the range of motion of their neck, which is often limited to about 10 degrees of movement. My second goal is to have their neck moving more than 50 degrees within the next six visits (70 degrees is considered within normal range, but 50 degrees is more functional than what they typically start with after months of wearing a collar). If the patient is responding, as my past experience suggests they should, then their outcome should be as successful as my previous patients with similar injuries.

The bonus of seeing a chiropractor is that even if your condition can't be helped by manual therapy, we can offer advice on alternative treatments like herbs, better nutrition, and other self-care options specific to your condition. In these ways, chiropractors supplement your medical care (if not negate your need for additional care).

If people are going to spend their health dollars on a treatment, that treatment should have a favorable outcome. To help determine whether progress is being made, measurements should be taken incrementally during the course of the treatments to show objectively whether the patient is responding favorably. If there is no measurable improvement partway through the treatment, then the condition needs to be reexamined. You may be getting treatment for the wrong condition. You cannot keep doing the same treatment and expect a different result.

I have had multiple patients come see me after their previous chiropractor failed to make them feel better after dozens of treatments. I was glad these patients were willing to suspend blame on the tool of chiropractic. With my chiropractic skills, I was able to help them feel better after just a few treatments. The rare times I cannot help a patient, I direct them to health practitioners who can.

It is important to find a practitioner who is willing and able to be your partner in obtaining optimal health. That practitioner should know their limitations and whether the treatment options for you go beyond their abilities. If they are not willing to be your partner, they are unlikely to help you reach optimal health. When a practitioner reaches their limitation in being able to help you, that is their limitation, not necessarily your limitation on being able to get well.

Think of all the aliments that used to be considered untreatable. They were not truly untreatable, but instead were outside the abilities of medical care at the time. These same ailments *are* treatable today because of the increase in medical knowledge. Unfortunately, we healthcare providers may not know the treatment you need, even if a treatment is currently available for you.

It reminds me of the old joke, "Do you know what they call the person who graduated at the bottom of his class at medical school? Doctor." Just because one doctor or one type of healthcare practitioner cannot help you solve your problem does not mean your problem is unsolvable.

Is the Practitioner Open to Me Seeing Other Practitioners?

I always welcome other practitioners' views on my patients' wellness. Not just from specialists in other fields, but from other chiropractors as well. Everyone brings something unique to the table, and sometimes new eyes bring new perspectives. I have a dozen patients who see other chiropractors for treatments I do not offer or because the other chiropractor is more convenient (closer to their work or home); these patients see me only when their treatments are not helping as expected and they need another opinion. Some patients simply like to have a relationship with multiple chiropractors so they are more likely to be seen in a timely manner.

I encourage all of my patients to see a variety of other health practitioners (medical doctors, acupuncturists, massage therapists, physical therapists, etc.). At a minimum, these other practitioners confirm my diagnosis and treatments. If they do not confirm it, then it prompts me to reexamine the problem more deeply. This can provide a learning experience for me and further confirmation for the patient. Or the patient may have two different opinions and more information to bring to a third practitioner to find the root of the problem. In either case, the collaboration is more helpful than the Lone Ranger approach.

I cannot tell you how many times patients have come to me after seeing several doctors, each of whom gave the patient a different diagnosis. I examine the patient and review what has already been done so I can help them determine the root cause and they can figure out their next step toward wellness.

I have had health practitioners tell their patients not to see other practitioners. I have had several patients who were told by their physical therapists not to see me because seeing both a chiropractor and physical therapist was "the same thing" and that it would be "fraudulent" to bill insurance for two of the same treatments. I believe this is a sign of the other practitioner's own insecurities, not a sign of a practitioner who has your best interests at heart.

You have the right to see as many healing professionals as you need to in order to get to the core of your condition. Each type of practitioner (and maybe even each individual practitioner) will have their own individual technique to offer. If nothing else, they can help verify that you are receiving the right kind of treatment.

If you receive satisfactory answers to the first four questions, then after seeing the provider over time, ask yourself the following questions:

Is the Practitioner Actually Helping Me?

Do their treatments hurt? Some therapists have a "no pain, no gain" mentality, resulting in treatments that may be more painful than they need to be.

If you feel like your healthcare provider (be it massage or physical therapist, chiropractor, acupuncturist, or any other practitioner) is hurting you, even if they are not, your belief that they are hurting you will impair your healing. This phenomenon is called "the negative placebo effect."

I always tell my patients to listen to their instincts. If what I do or say does not jive with them, they should tell me. Their instinct always trumps my recommendation or technique. It just means we have to find another technique that works for them, both physically and mentally. You cannot separate the two.

Many of my patients say that, for such a small female, I give a mighty adjustment and dig deep with my soft-tissue work. But many patients receive ultra-gentle care from me. I cater my treatment to the patient's needs and limitations. I am not going to adjust a construction worker the same as I would an elderly lady with osteopenia.

There are times where I am pressing on tender muscles, but I aim to produce good pain. My patients understand that it may hurt in the moment, but the body knows it is a good hurt and a productive movement toward wellness. I never want to cause bad pain. That, to me, is a pressure that causes more harm than good, such as bruising healthy tissues. I aim to mobilize joints, not strain them.

This is where the art of practice comes into play. Anyone can move a joint, but not everyone can move it safely and well in a manner that that patient is comfortable with. That is why such practices take years of education and require licensure.

If you have had a rough chiropractic experience, I hope you recognize that it was the practitioner and not the tool that caused your negative experience, and give chiropractic a second (more educated) chance.

Is the Practitioner Living Up to My Expectations?

At your first appointment, a practitioner should give you a rough timeline of when you should start seeing results, how likely you will recover, and to what degree. If you are not seeing the results as expected, get another opinion. Do not be afraid to seek more than one healer's advice to validate the root cause of your pain.

When a patient isn't seeing results as expected, it can be due to the provider not treating you completely or a misdiagnosis resulting in the wrong treatment being prescribed.

My least favorite thing is when a patient comes in with what I call a "garbage can diagnosis," which is basically a fancy combination of Latin words that describe their symptoms but not any underlying causes or conditions. Then, armed with this "diagnosis," a medical doctor will generally attempt to cover up the patient's symptoms with drugs. It is relatively easy to do, and everyone is happy at the cessation of symptoms. But the long-term cost of this approach is immeasurable: The patient's health will continue to deteriorate over time because no one is addressing the root of the problem.

To make matters worse, the effectiveness of any medicine decreases over time as the body learns to break it down. This reduced effectiveness results in having to increase the dose over time. Sadly, the patient is trained to blame this problem on the fact that they are aging. No! The patient needs to learn what the root of the problem is so they can properly treat it and so their body can start healing over time instead of worsening.

I love my job. Every day I get to watch people transform from the belief that their health was naturally going to worsen with time to a place where their lives and abilities actually *improve* over time. I have many patients who are healthier in their forties and fifties than they were in their twenties and thirties.

Does Every Visit Have the Same Treatment?

The first few visits may be the same because you are in acute pain. But as you improve, your treatments should evolve. You should transition from passive, palliative treatments, like gentle mobilization and electrical muscle stimulation, to more active care, like muscle strengthening, and self-care management. Your practitioner should give you instructions on how to strengthen your weak and injured muscles and stretch your tight and spastic protective muscles in between visits to their office.

Healthcare when mapped out for your specific needs (versus a cookie-cutter format) will shorten your pathway to wellness.

Good luck creating your optimal healing team!

Triad of Wellness

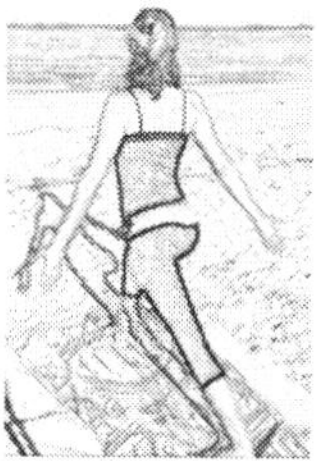

Sleep & Think Well

Relax & meditate
to rest and take the
"weight off your shoulders."

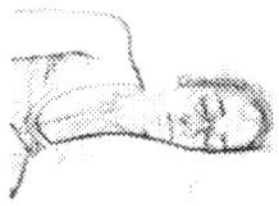

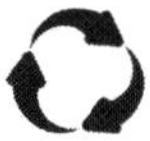

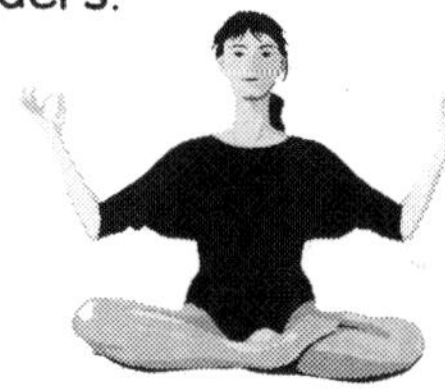

Exercise & Stretch Well

Check your posture. Stretch and
strengthen to have the means to
hold up your heavy head.
Invert frequently to take the
physical pressure off your neck.

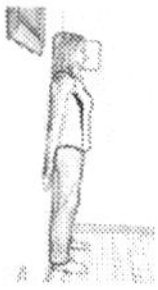

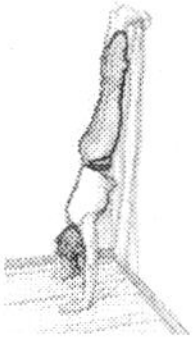

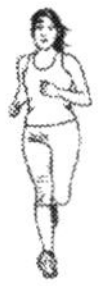

Eat & Hydrate Well

To provide nutrients to every
cell in your body, so they can
function, repair and live!

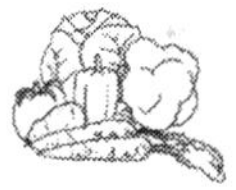

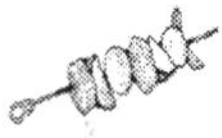

In Conclusion . . .

If your neck pain is not due to some underlying disease, using some, if not all, of the techniques I've included in this book should reduce or eliminate the need to take pain-relieving medication. On the rare occasion you still need a pain pill or shot, it should work even better for you because your body will not have built up a tolerance to the remedy.

I hope this book has been informative and will enable you to be more collaborative with your professional healthcare providers so you can plan your path to a pain-free and healthy life.

If I have helped you, I have fulfilled my mission in writing this book. I am writing my Combat Dis-Ease Series—each book a message in a bottle I send out in a sea of confusing and conflicting information—with the hope that the books provide information that helps you find your way to wellness.

Please help me help others by sharing this book and writing a review on Amazon to encourage others to read this book.

Wishing you the best of health,

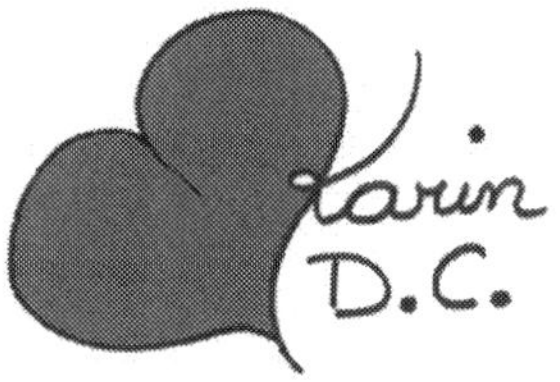

Karin Drummond, DC

Quick Reference for Basic Trigger Points, Pressure Points, Stretches, and Exercises for Neck Pain

Figures in Chapter 9

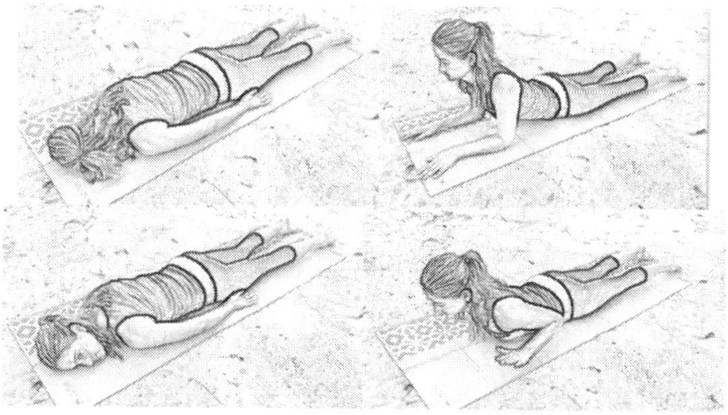

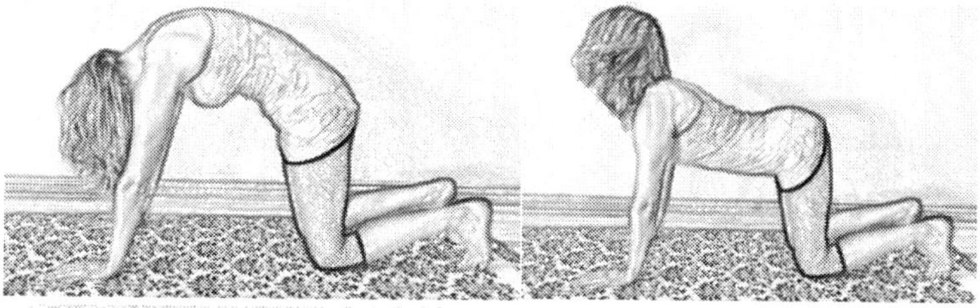

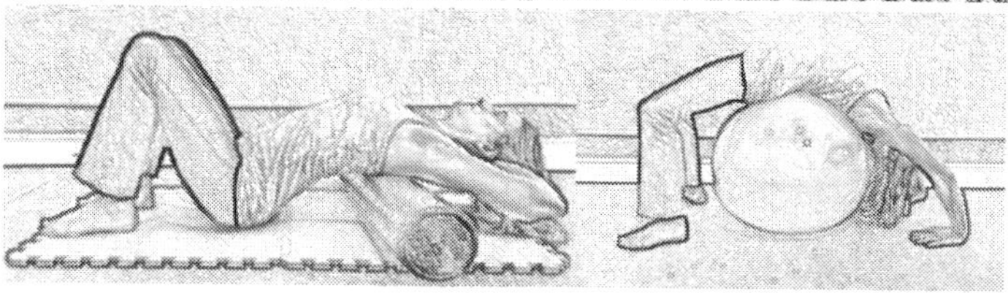

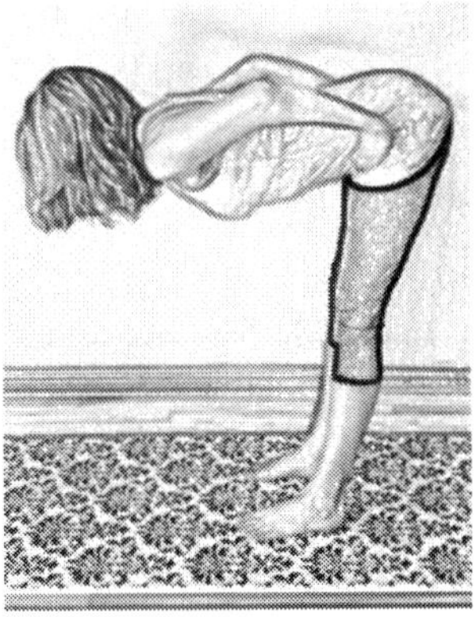

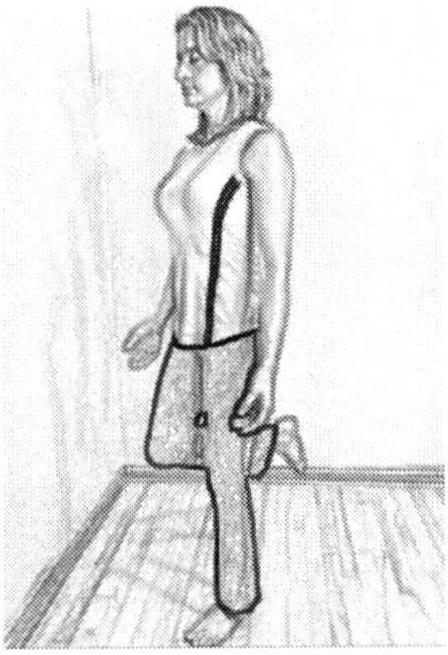

Figures in Chapter 10

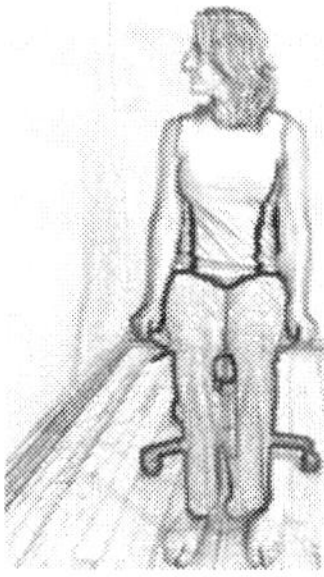
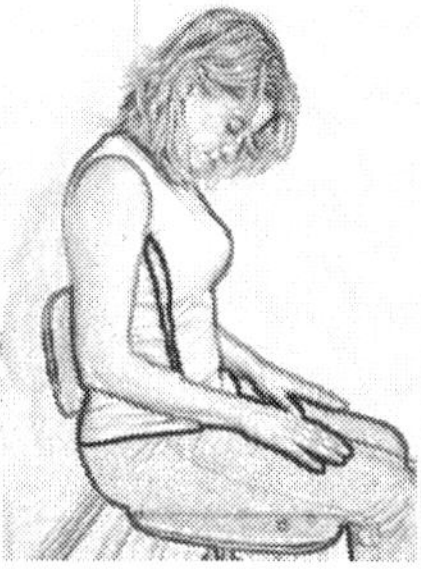
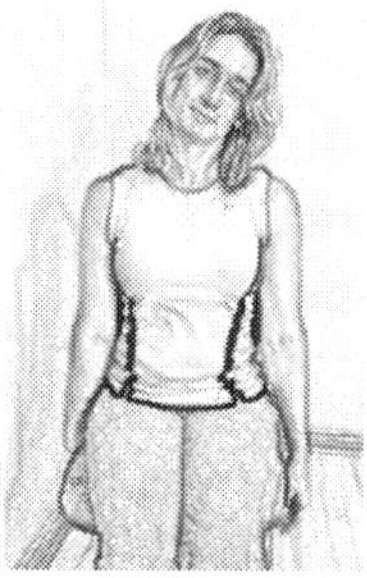
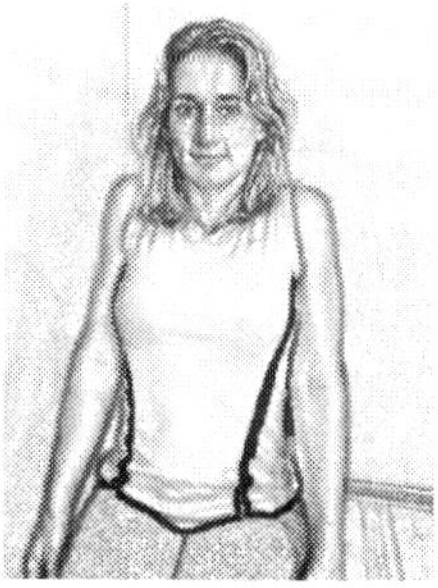
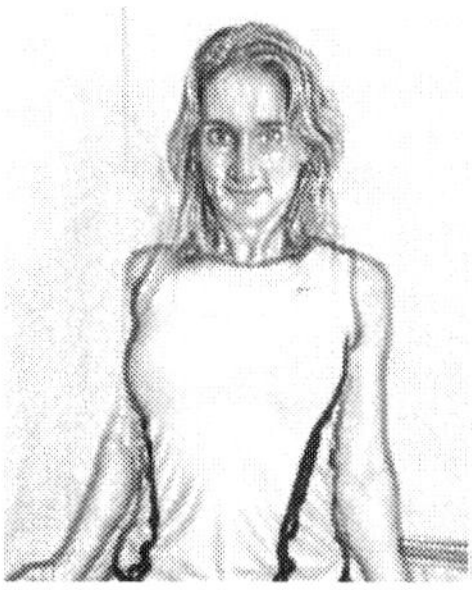
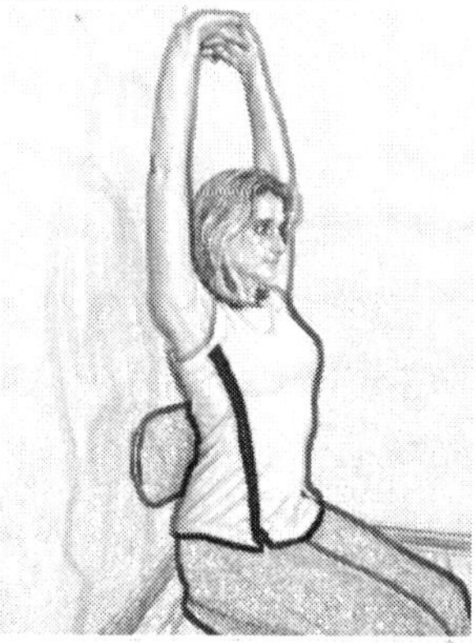
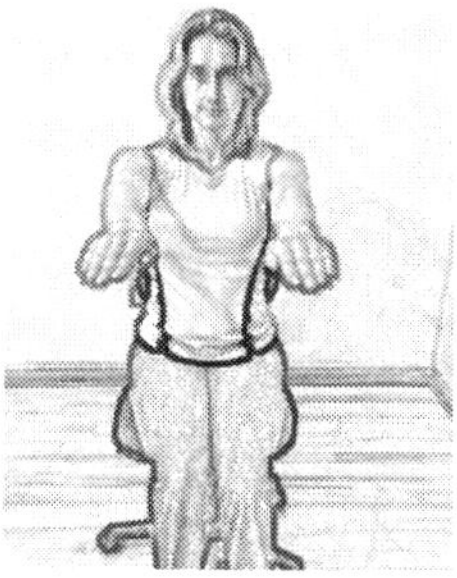
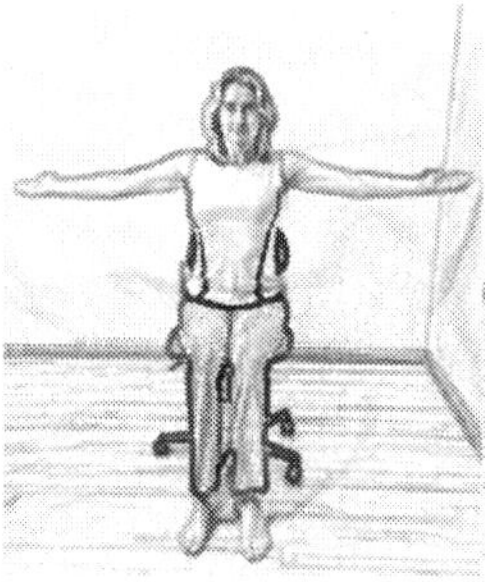
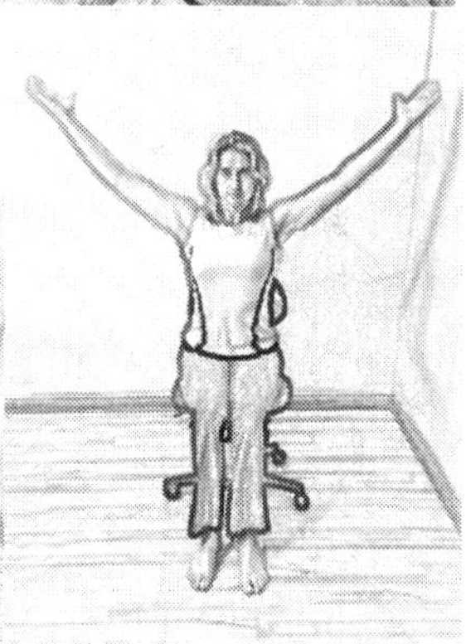

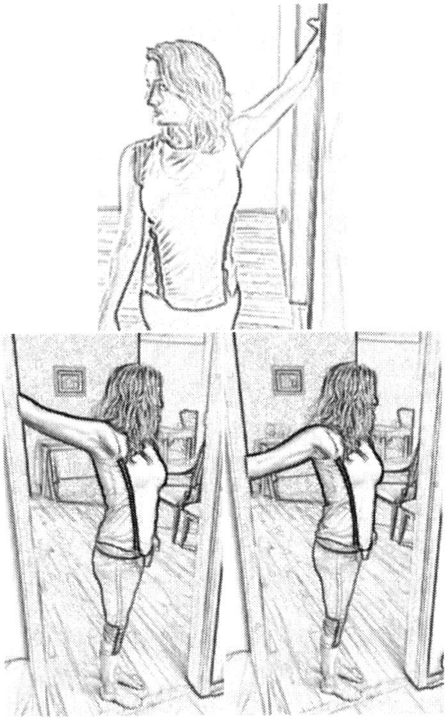

Figures in Chapter 11

Neck isometrics

Neck Post-Isometric Stretches

Rotation

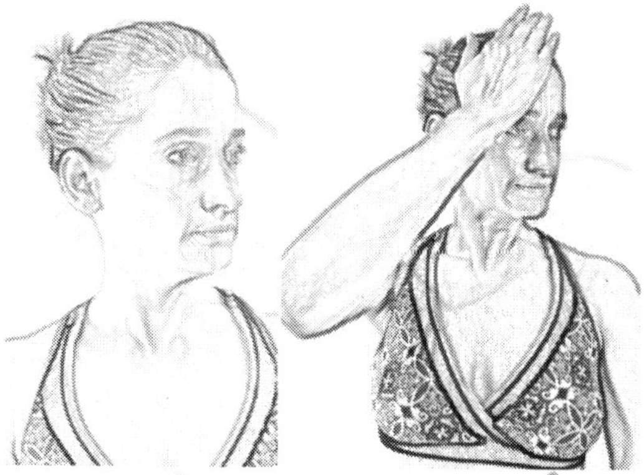

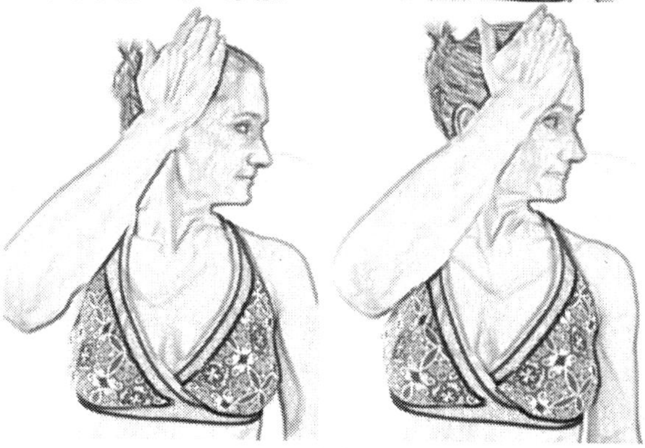

Lateral flexion

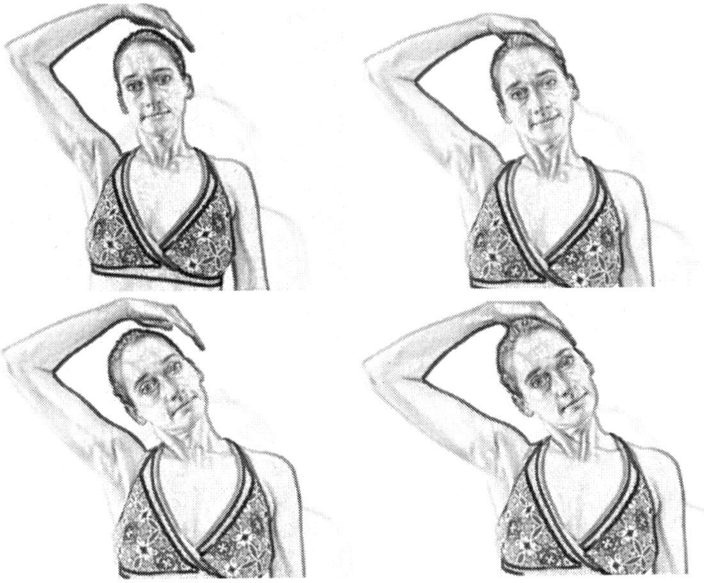

Posterior neck isometric

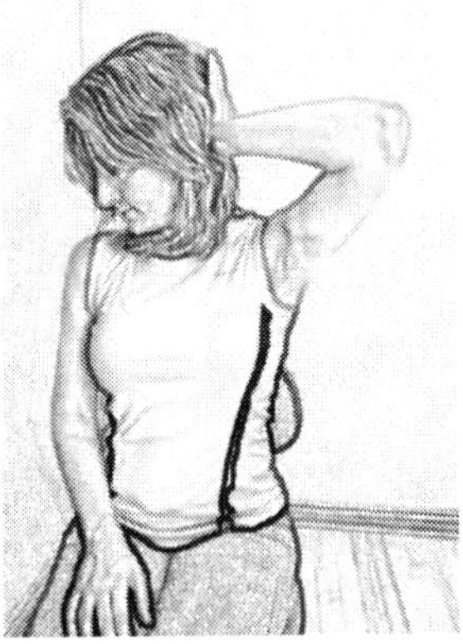

Rhomboid exercises

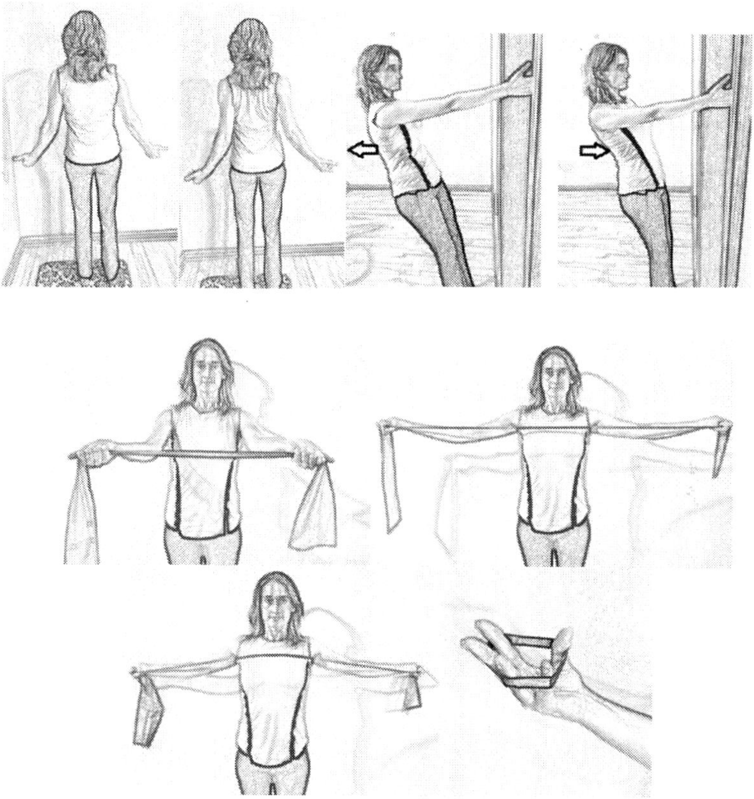

Figures in Chapter 12

Abdominal workout

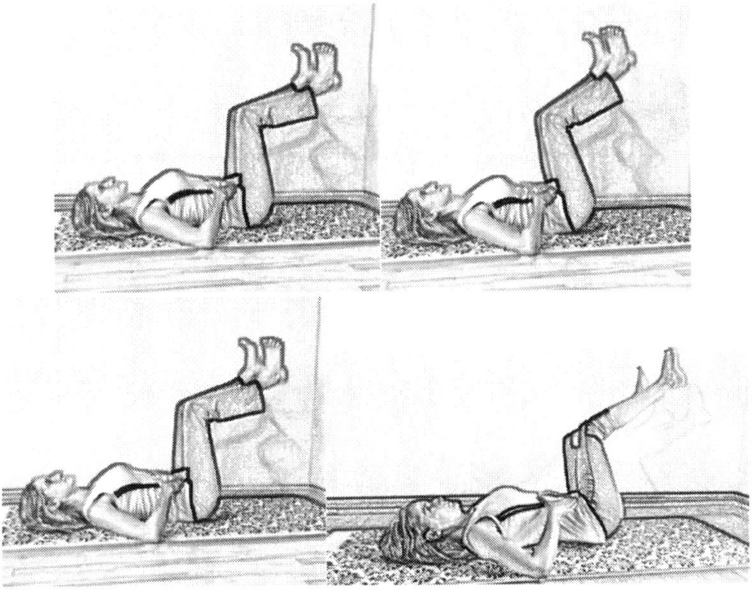

Abdominal stretch (thigh exercise)

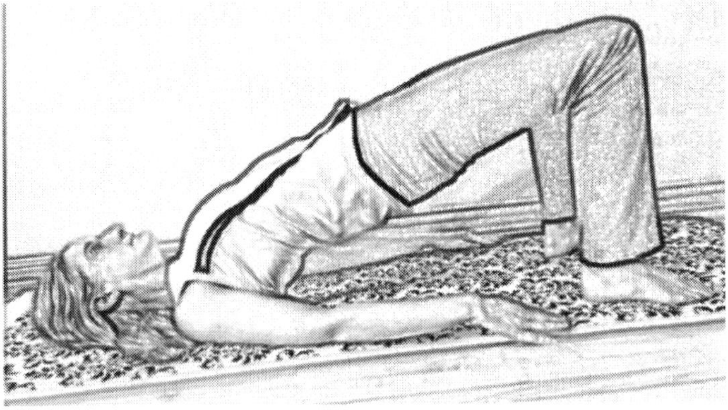

Figures in Chapter 13

Self-massage

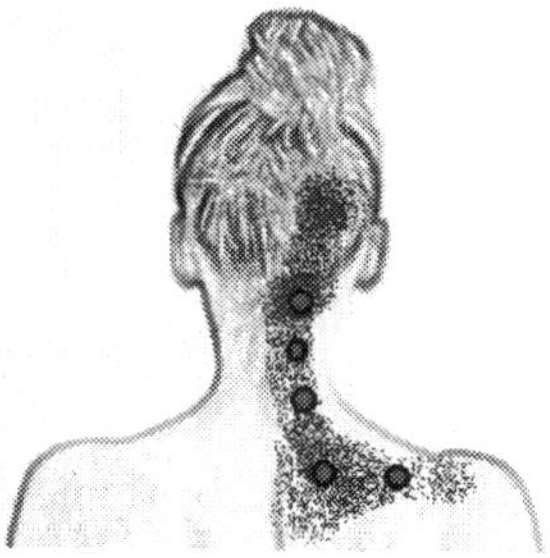

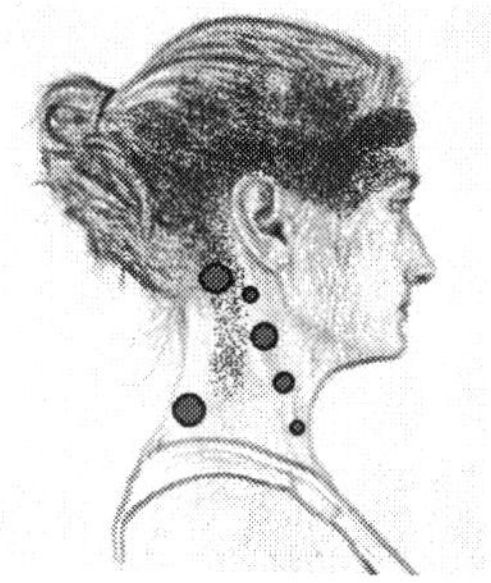

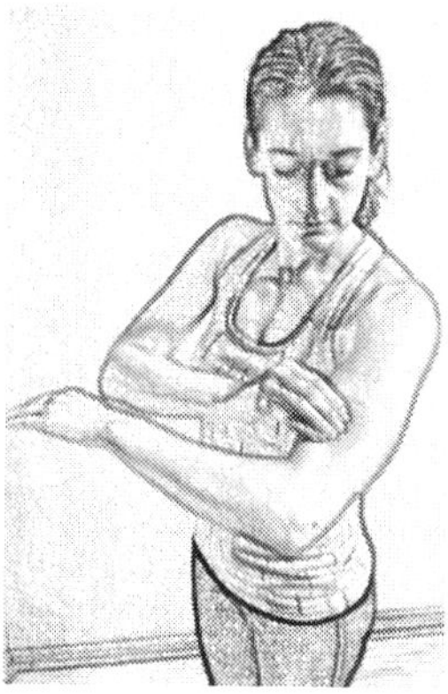

REFERENCES

American Gastroenterological Association. "Study Shows Long-term Use of NSAIDs Causes Severe Intestinal Damage." ScienceDaily. www.sciencedaily.com/releases/2005/01/050111123706.htm.

Astin, J.A. and E. Ernst. "The Effectiveness of Spinal Manipulation for the Treatment of Headache Disorders: A systematic review of randomized clinical trials." *Cephalalgia* 22, no. 8 (2002): 617–623.

Blower, A., A. Brooks, C.G. Fenn, A. Hill, M.Y. Pearce, S. Morant, and K.D. Bardhan. "Emergency Admissions for Upper Gastrointestinal Disease and Their Relation to NSAIDs Use." *Alimentary Pharmacology and Therapeutics* 11, no. 2 (1997): 283–91.

Bronfort, G., R. Evans, A.V. Anderson, K.H. Svendsen, Y. Bracha, and R.H. Grimm. "Spinal Manipulation, Medication, or Home Exercise with Advice for Acute and Subacute Neck Pain: A Randomized Trial." *Annals of Internal Medicine* 156 (2012): 1-10. doi:10.7326/0003-4819-156-1-201201030-00002.

Bryans, R., M. Descarreaux M, Duranleau, H. Marcoux, B. Potter, R. Ruegg, L. Shaw, R. Watkin, and E. White. "Evidence-based Guidelines for the Chiropractic Treatment of Adults with Headache." *Journal of Manipulative and Physiological Therapeutics* 34, no. 5 (June 2011): 274-89. doi:10.1016/j.jmpt.2011.04.008.

Cassidy, J.D., E. Boyle, P. Côté, Y. He, S. Hogg-Johnson, F.L. Silver, and S.J. Bondy. "Risk of Vertebrobasilar Stroke and Chiropractic Care: Results of a Population-Based Case-Control and Case-Crossover Study." *Spine* 33 (4 Suppl) (2008): S176–183.

Fries, J.F., S.R. Miller, P.W. Spitz, C.A Williams, H.B. Hubert, and D.A. Bloch. "Toward an Epidemiology of Gastropathy

Associated with Nonsteroidal Anti-inflammatory Drug Use." *Gastroenterology* 96 (1989): 647–655.

Jensen. P. Your Chiropractic Wellness (blog). "Chiropractic Education vs. Medical Education." http://yourchiropracticwellness.com/tag/chiropractic-education-vs-medical-education.

Mayo Clinic. "Chiropractic Adjustment." Last updated August 13, 2015. www.mayoclinic.org/tests-procedures/chiropractic-adjustment/basics/risks/prc-20013239.

National Weather Service. "How Dangerous is Lightning?" www.lightningsafety.noaa.gov/odds.shtml.

Ruiz-Torres, A. and W. Beier. "On Maximum Human Life Span: Interdisciplinary approach about its limits." *Advances in Gerontology* 16 (2005): 14–20. www.ncbi.nlm.nih.gov/pubmed/16075672.

Stone, J.A.M. and Johnstone, P.A.S. "Mechanisms of Action for Acupuncture in the Oncology Setting." *Current Treatment Options in Oncology* 11, no. 3 (2010): 118–127. doi:10.1007/s11864-010-0128-y.

Vicodin Addiction. "Nearly 100 Percent of the World's Vicodin Prescriptions Are Used in U.S." www.addictionvicodin.com/addiction-news/all-the-worlds-vicodin-prescriptions-in-united-states/.

Williams, S., C. Whatman, P.A. Hume, and K. Sheerin. "Kinesio Taping in Treatment and Prevention of Sports Injuries: A Meta-Analysis of the Evidence for its Effectiveness." *Sports Medicine* 42, no. 2 (February 2012): 153–164. doi:10.2165/11594960-000000000-00000.

World Health Organization. "Acupuncture: Review and Analysis of Reports on Controlled Clinical Trials." http://apps.who.int/medicinedocs/pdf/s4926e/s4926e.pdf.

Zimmerman, H.J. "Drugs Used to Treat Rheumatic and Musculospastic Disease." In *Hepatotoxicity: The Adverse Effects of Drugs and Other Chemicals on the Liver*, 2nd ed. Philadelphia: Lippincott, 1999, 517–553.

ABOUT THE AUTHOR

Karin Drummond, DC, lives in Bloomington, Indiana. She graduated with distinction from the University of Victoria with a bachelor of science degree. She finished the four-year doctorate of chiropractic degree at the University of Western States in 2000. She moved to her husband's hometown of Bloomington, Indiana, and has practiced there ever since. She now calls it home, living at its edge in the country with her husband and two children. She has been voted her town's number-one chiropractor seven times as of 2016.

Passionate about living well, she keeps up with new research in the health field and practices what she preaches. Her patients have told her for years that she needed to write a book because she is such a great source of information on healthy living. Once she discovered how easy it was to publish a book, she decided to take advantage of this medium to help spread her thoughts on living well. Her first book, *Top Seven Ways to Combat the Effects of Sitting,* was published in 2015 and was a finalist in the 2016 Best Book Awards in the Health – Diet and Exercise category. She has published several books since then, and she is planning on publishing many more books on a variety of topics.

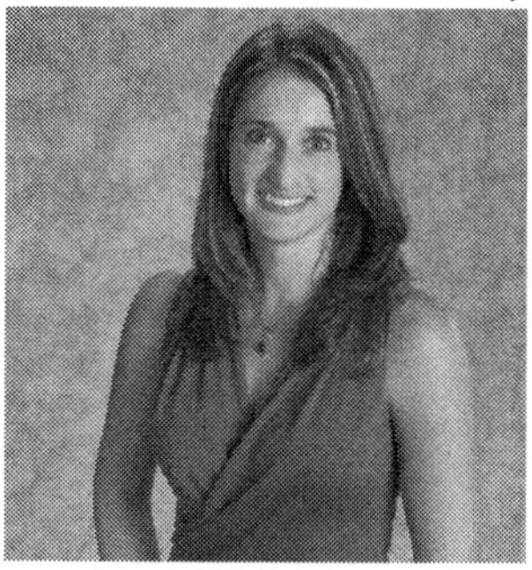

www.drkarindc.com

Other Books by Dr. Karin Drummond

Available now:

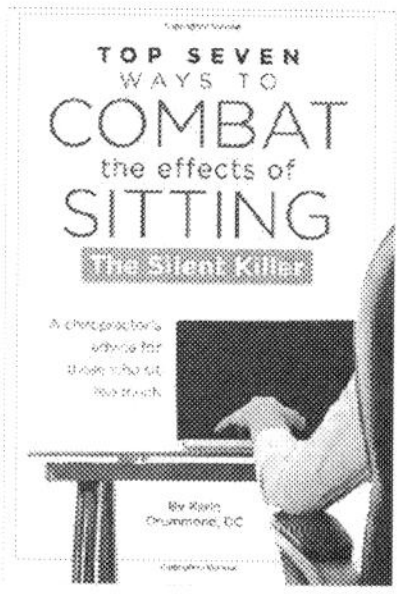

Top Seven Ways to Combat the Effects of Sitting: The Silent Killer

Finalist in the Best Book Awards in 2016 in the Health: Diet and Exercise category. It's a must read for those who sit too much.

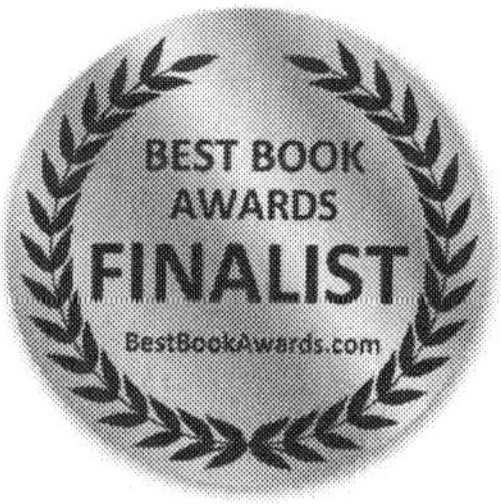

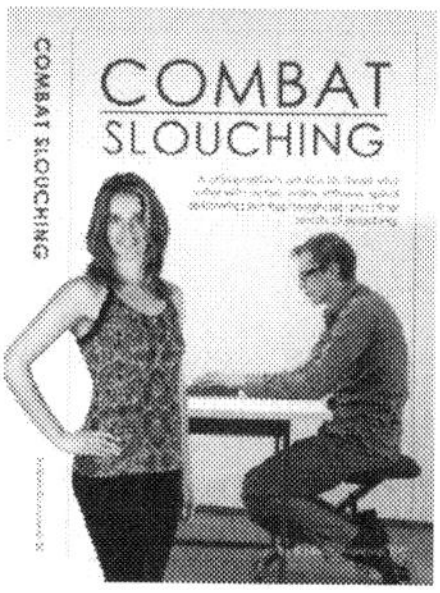

Combat Slouching

For those who suffer from aches, pains, stiffness, spinal deformities like hyperkyphosis, and other effects of slouching.

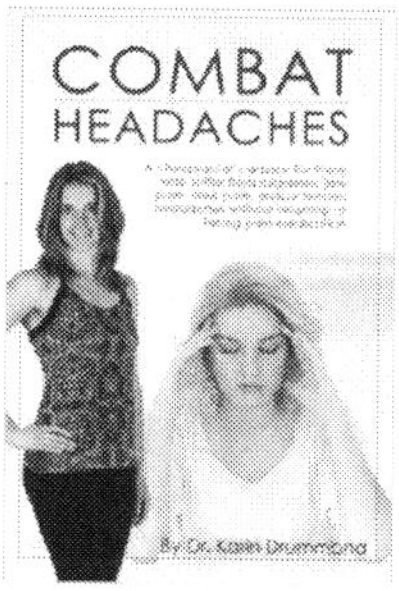

Combat Headaches

For those who suffer from migraines, jaw pain, sinus pain, and/or tension headaches without resorting to taking pain medication.

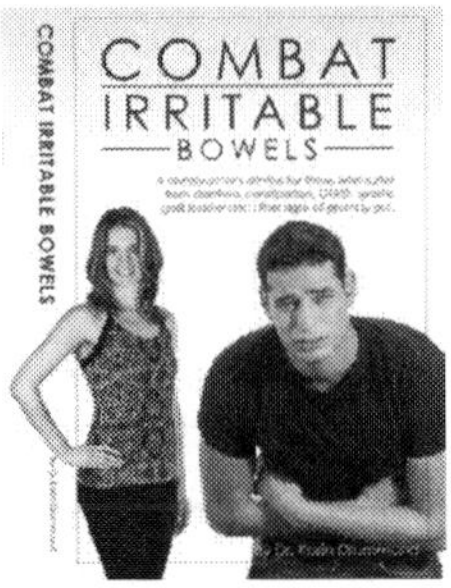

Combat Irritable Bowels

For those who suffer from diarrhea, constipation, spastic gallbladder, inflammation of the bowels, and other causes of abdominal pain.

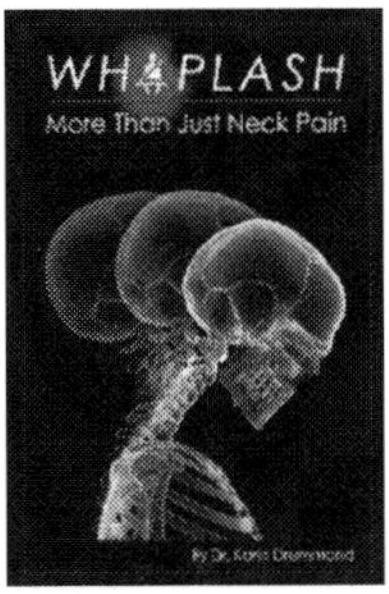

Whiplash: More Than Just Neck Pain

This booklet explains some of the mechanisms of whiplash and symptoms to watch out for.

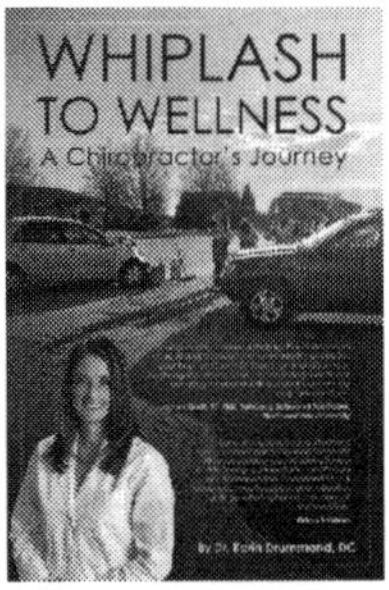

Whiplash to Wellness: A Chiropractor's Journey

The whiplash patient can easily relate to Dr. Karin Drummond's denial of the severity of symptoms and the frustration of daily life after this type of injury. We benefit from her journey as she shares her gems of knowledge. In true Dr. Drummond fashion, she speaks to us with compassion and knowledge, and educates us on modalities of recovery. –**Dr. Lisa Robinson, MD, Joie de Vivre Medical**

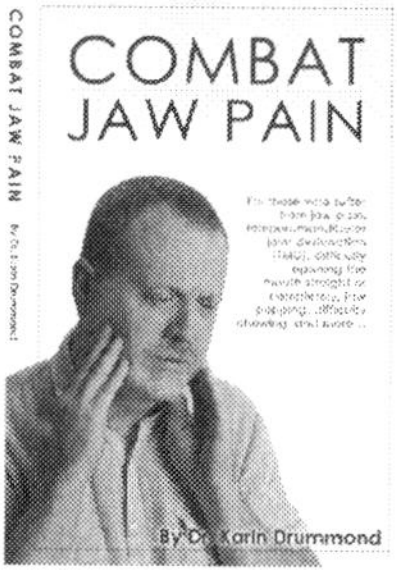

Combat Jaw Pain

For those who suffer with jaw pain, Temporomandibular Joint Dysfunction (TMD), difficulty opening the mouth straight or completely, jaw popping, difficulty chewing, and more…

Coming soon:

Combat Low Back Pain

Combat Foot Pain

and many other books …

All to help you find your personal path to wellness.

To find out more, visit Dr. Karin's website:
www.drkarindc.com

68036055R00137

Made in the USA
Lexington, KY
29 September 2017